RODENTS FOR PHARMACOLOGICAL EXPERIMENTS

RODENTS FOR PHARMACOLOGICAL EXPERIMENTS

Dr. TAPAN KUMAR CHATTERJEE
M.Pharm., FIC, Ph.D
Ex UGC Research Scientist,
Associate Professor,
Division of Pharmacology,
Department of Pharmaceutical Technology,
Jadavpur University, Kolkata-700032

PharmaMed Press
An imprint of Pharma Book Syndicate
A Unit of BSP Books Pvt. Ltd.
4-4-316, Giriraj Lane,
Sultan Bazar, Hyderabad - 500 095.

Published by

PharmaMed Press

An imprint of Pharma Book Syndicate

A Unit of BSP Books Pvt. Ltd.

4-4-309/316, Giriraj Lane, Sultan Bazar, Hyderabad - 500 095.

Phone: 040-23445605, 23445688; Fax: 91+40-23445611

E-mail: info@pharmamedpress.com

ISBN: 978-93-85433-51-1 (HB)

Dedicated to

My Parents

PREFACE

When I was on the career of study and research work, I confess that I badly needed the aid of a handbook on laboratory rodents for experimental references etc. I have, therefore, been motivated to compile this handbook to deliver substantial help to researchers who might be interested to carry on the research work on mice and rats.

This versatile compilation is the outcome of enlightening experiences, gained in course of my painstaking prolonged pharmacological research work, while I have in fact, extensively handled two laboratory rodents one relates to tiny mouse and the other to rat.

This assemblage would obviously create interests to those researchers, who are in quest of new pharmacologically active drugs. A variety of investigators in the field of pharmaceutics, physiology, pharmacognosy, toxicology may find useful information and data for their research works.

I myself experienced difficulties initially as a student and later as a researcher in the laboratory on the score of finding out the best way of handling laboratory mice and rats. On being goaded by the requests of many students and researchers for a comprehensive book on this subject. I made this venture to write the book entitled ***"Rodents for Pharmacological Experiments".*** This book has suit to publication within a short span of time , being compiled during my busy hours and it is not unlikely that the readers may notice some printing devil etc. and I sincerely hope that they shall bear with me on this count, in view of the unavoidable circumstances.

Section A of this book comprises about care, breeding, handling and nutrition etc. of laboratory mice and rats. And *Section B* assembles most important methods for screening pharmacologically active substances using mice and rats. While writing this book I have made efforts to collect the simplest and most widely used screening methods. Absolute completeness has not yet been attempt. The methods here are thoroughly and vividly written, thus providing readers with up-to date information.

For compilation of the salient materials of this handbook I am indebted to the authors of various books and leading laboratory data written on animals.

It would have been impossible to complete this hand book without the invaluable assistance of Mr Hariome Singh, Mr Saumen Karan, Mr Saswata Banerjee, Mr Biswajit Das and Mr Souvik Debnath who kindly laid hands in correction of the manuscript and helped in preparation of sketches. I must thanks them for all assistance rendered to me in this venture.

Handbook is the result of enormous encouragement received from my family. Moral support of my wife and daughter have been a fortunate thing for writing this book. My father (who wrote more than 80 informative article in journals) is one of my role models as an author.

I am grateful to my publisher "BSP Books Pvt.Ltd." and to their editorial staff for their co-operation, encouragement and valuable suggestions. I hope the handbook will be useful for the students, researchers and teachers. Suggestion and comments are always welcome from any part.

It is a handbook to read, keep and refer to again and again.

Kolkata- 700032
March, 2013

Dr. T.K. Chatterjee

CONTENTS

INTRODUCTION

Rodentia is the order of mammals known as **rodents**, characterized by a single pair of incessantly growing incisors in each of the upper and lower jaws which must be kept diminutive by gnawing.

Forty percent of mammal species are rodents, and they are found in immense numbers on all continents other than Antarctica. Common rodents include mice, rats, squirrels, porcupines, beavers, guinea pigs, and hamsters. Rodents use their sharp incisors to gnaw wood, break into food, and bite predators. Most rodents consume seeds or plants, though some have more assorted diets. Some species have traditionally been pests, ingesting seeds stored by people and scattering disease.

In terms of number of species—although not inevitably in terms of number of organisms (population) or biomass—rodents make up the largest order of mammals. With about 2,277 species of rodents, over 40% of mammalian species belong to the order. Their success is probably due to their small size, short breeding cycle, and ability to gnaw and consume a wide variety of foods.

Members of non-rodent orders, such as Chiroptera (bats), Scandentia (treeshrews), Soricomorpha (shrews and moles), Lagomorpha (hares, rabbits and pikas) and mustelid carnivores such as weasels and mink, are sometimes confused with rodents.

Rodents are set up in vast numbers on all continents except Antarctica, most islands, and in all habitats except oceans. They are the only nonvolant, non-marine placental norder—and in particular are the only placental order besides bats and pinnipeds—to have reached Australia without human introduction.

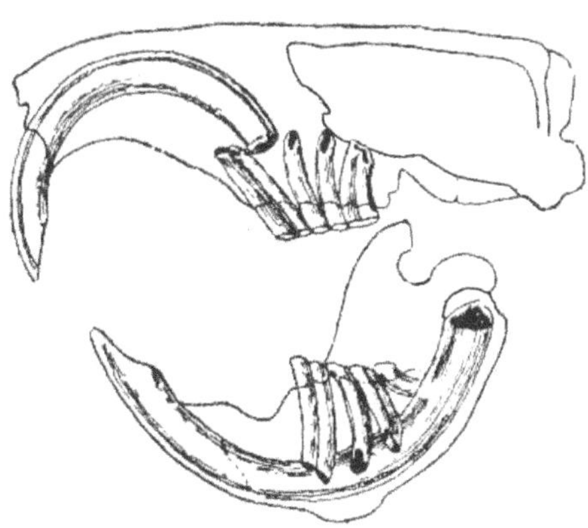

Fig. Typical rodent tooth system.

Practically all rodents contribute to the characteristic of dentition extremely expert for gnawing. This specialization gives rodents their name from the Latin, *rodere*, to gnaw. All rodents, except *Paucidentomys vermidax*, have a single pair of upper and a single pair of lower incisors followed by a gap (diastema), and then one or more molars or premolars; *Paucidentomys vermidax* is unique among the rodents in that it possesses no molars or premolars, and its incisors are so dedicated, they are not for gnawing.

Owing to the wide multiplicity of their characteristics, some of which are considered uncommon or unique amongst mammals, rodents are used widely in research. For example, the naked mole rat, *Heterocephalus glaber,* is the only known mammal that is poikilothermic and also does not produce the neurotransmitter substance P; it is therefore used in studies on thermoregulation and pain.

Oftentimes mice experiments are done to know something about what happens to humans, and it boils down to assuming that certain bodily processes in mice are the same as in humans, or at least similar enough to illustrate conclusions by analogy, e.g. how mice and men react to poisonous substances. Not all processes are analogous - for example, mouse and human brains are amply different that other animals (monkeys, apes, etc) are used.

There is also a combined effect, in that once many experiments on mice are done, more data are available about the validity of the animal model, thus making further experiments on mice easier to understand since scientists recognize more about how good a model a mouse is for some meticulous biological process in humans.

In this present book, two types of rodent (**Mice & Rats**) are included for pharmacological experiments.

White mice are the least laboratory animals that can be bred consistently, are cheap and effortless to handle, and being very small are sensitive to small doses of a substance. Swiss albino mouse is the most widely used strain for laboratory investigations.

Mice are employed extensively in acute toxicity studies. They are also used for the assay of insulin and analgesics, the latter specially against chemically induced pain. General screening of chemotherapeutic agents is undertaken in this species. Specially bred mice are used for the study of the problems in genetics and in cancer research. Mice are most frequently used for the testing of drugs for teratogenicity. The development of nude mouse, a hairless genetic mutant that lacks a thymus, and thus deficeient in T lymphocytes, has been of fundamental interest in the field of tissue immunity and transplantation research. Albino rat is one of the commonest laboratory animals appropriate for experimental work because of its small size and greater sensitivity to most drugs. It is also the most consistent of all laboratory animals. It can be bred to acquire unadulterated and homogeneous strains, and is found to be very well-built to endure long periods of experimentation under anesthesia.

There are two original strains of albino rats, *Wistar* and *Sprague-Dawley* that have been extensively used all the way through the world.

Wistar rat is a quiet, reasonably prolific strain quite resistant to infection, and has low incidence of spontaneous tumours. The head is wide, especially in the male, and the ears are long. The tail-length is always less than the body-length.

Sprague-Dawley rat is more speedily growing and more prolific than Wistar rat, and has a longer and narrower head, and a longer tail, which may equal the body-length. It is also less resistant to infection, specially to respiratory disease.

There are certain anatomical peculiarities that should be distinguished. Rodents do not vomit because they be deficient in vomiting centre. Rats do not have any tonsil or a gall bladder.

SECTION-A

GENERAL DISCUSSION ABOUT LABORATORY MICE AND RATS

This part of the book envisages fundamental knowledge on handling, housing, breeding, nutrition etc. of laboratory mice and rats. Handling involves two most important responsibilities on the part of experimenters. These responsibilities are primarily a most scrupulous care to the effect that the animals suffer no pain and secondly a sincere regard for the health and well-being of the animal colony. As for the well-being of the colony, the experimenters should assume much of the responsibility. This is not pure caretaker work. They should take pride in visual appearance of the animal colony, in having sleek, well-nourished animals in clean sanitary lodgings. Familarity with their habits, demeanours and care for their well-being will enrich dividends, in a minor way in a reduced incidence of animal bites and in a major way in an increased incidence of successful results in pharmacology research.

This section also includes some important biological and physiological data of laboratory mice and rats in tabular form.

The Laboratory Mouse▲

CLASS : Mammalia ORDER : Rodentia

FAMILY: Murinae

SCIENTIFIC NAME: *Mus musculus*

Amongst all animals used in the laboratory experiments the mouse is considered as the most widely used one which is, available for use all over the world. To sort out number of research problems, mouse stands as the animal of choice, because of its tiny size, early sexual maturity (puberty), high fecundity (fertility), short gestation period (length of time from conception to birth) as well as relatively higher position in the evolutionary scale. In the field of laboratory tests, about millions of mice are used all over the world in a year. In the field of cancer research, reproductive biology, diagnosis, study of drug, screening, immunology, toxicology and genetics, numerous variety of inbred strains of mice are available for being profusely used.

The Swiss albino mouse has been selected here as the representative of the species for resume of discussions herein, this animal being most popular amongst the numerous inbred strains available.

Exterior Features of Mouse

The body of the mouse is slender with smooth hair-coat, long pointed snout, prominent round ears and long flat front sharp teeth. The average weight of an adult mouse is about 30 gms. and the length is about 7.5 cm. from snout to the base of tail. The tail is hairless. The female mouse has five pairs of nipples, three pairs on the thoracic region and two pairs on the abdominal region.

Anatomical Peculiarities of Mouse

Like other rodents, in mice a single pair of upper incisors are present. The incisors are chisel-shaped in wear owing to the absence of enamel on their posterior surfaces and having persistently open roots. They grow throughout life and are always of great size. Canines are never present, and there is wide diastema between the incisors and cheek-teeth into which the cheeks can be tucked so as to separate the front part of the mouth from the hind during the process of gnawing. An adaptation of the jaws enables the animal for gnawing. The grinding-teeth vary in number and frequently have persistently open roofs. To provide the necessary power for gnawing. The jaw-muscles are very greatly enlarged. The brain of mouse is little, convoluted and the cerebellum is not covered by the cerebral lobes. The sternum of the mice has a long and narrow body. The skull is elongated narrow in front, broader and depressed behind. The nasal cavities are very large, with complex air sinuses in their upper part. The orbit and temporal fossa are continuous. A remarkable feature of the skull is the presence of many large opening corresponding to the infraorbital foramen. The bones of the arm and forearm show considerable variation. In the alimentary canal there is large caecum. The placenta is duciduate. The mice do not vomit because they lack vomiting centre [absence of CTZ].

Housing of Mouse

Normally in animal house, mice are housed in the cages of shoebox type, made of plastic, galvanised iron, anodized, aluminium or stainless steel and the floor of such cages may be either screen bottomed or solid. The screen bottom cages are always suspended and the solid bottom cages may either be suspended or standing on a rack. In case of screen bottom (wire mesh) cages, the diameter of the wire and the mesh size should be appropriate to afford maximum comfort to the living animal housed on it. A floor mesh (grid) size of 3 × 3 openings per inch being made of 18 guage (0.0475 inch) wire is ideal for housing mice. A tray is placed at the bottom of the cages when screen bottom cages are in use, for the purpose of collecting urine and faeces droppings, Usually, some materials are provided as bedding in solid bottom cages as such bedding would absorb urine and moisture from faeces. It also aids comfort to the animal. For such bedding, rice husk are used widely. The size of the cage of animals, should commensurate with the age and number of animals to be housed in the cage and the minimum floor space should be 97 sq. cm. per adult mouse. The minimum height of the cage should be 12.7 cm, (5.0 inch). Housing in a cage in groups for weanings or adult females is possible; but housing of adult males in groups will create bitter fighting pell-mell in the cage. Maximum housing number of mice in a cage must not exceed 20. A cage with dimensions of 25 × 20 × 15 cm^3 will comfortably bear either a pair (a male and a female) or one male with two females with litters (the young brought forth at a birth) or six adult mice.

Requirement of External Environment for Mouse

The temperature of the mouse-housing room may be maintained any where in the range of 20-25°C. An optimal temperature for the mouse is 22 ±1°C. The relative humidity (RH) should be held between 45% and 55%. Twelve to fifteen changes of air per hour in the animal room, are recommended. Lighting and darkness be divided in equal number of hours viz 12 hours of lighting and 12 hours of darkness, which should be provided in the room for optimal growth and reproduction. Intensity of light inside the animal room should be between 350- 400 lux one meter above the level of floor. Mice are very sensitive to noise particularly in the midst of higher- frequencies of human auditory range and beyond it ; hence noisy atmosphere has to be eliminated to the maximum for healthy living of mice.

Nutritional Requirement of Mouse

Laboratory mice are fed either with commercially available pellet diet or diet formulated in the animal facilities. By use of a variety of cereals, pulses, seeds etc. the diet can be formulated for use. In order to ensure proper growth and reproduction, mice should be fed on stock diet containing 16 – 25% protein, 4 – 6% fat, and 45 – 55% carbohydrate. In addition, normal diet should contain all the major vitamins in definite proportions and essential minerals in specific quantities. The diet should be tasty to the animal and one which can be easily formulated and stored conveniently. An adult mouse normally consumes 4 to 5 gms. of diet per day. The consumption of daily diet of animal varies depending on the physiological status of the animal as well as environmental temperature. Food consumption, increases considerably in the pregnancy or lactating stage of animal. Clear water should be provided to the animal for drinking *ad libitum.* An adult mouse drinks about 6 ml. of water per day.

Handling of Mouse

Mice are by nature very timid, social, nocturnal and escape prone rodents. Mouse can be picked up by holding at the base of tail. The animal however, should not be caught by the tip of the tail, since it would cause severe pains to the animal. For the purpose of inspection on manipulations, the mouse is lifted by tail, placed on a rough "toe-gripping" surface, such as the top of a case, grasped on the scruff of the neck by thumb and forefinger. The animal is then inverted and the tail is held between the little finger and palm.

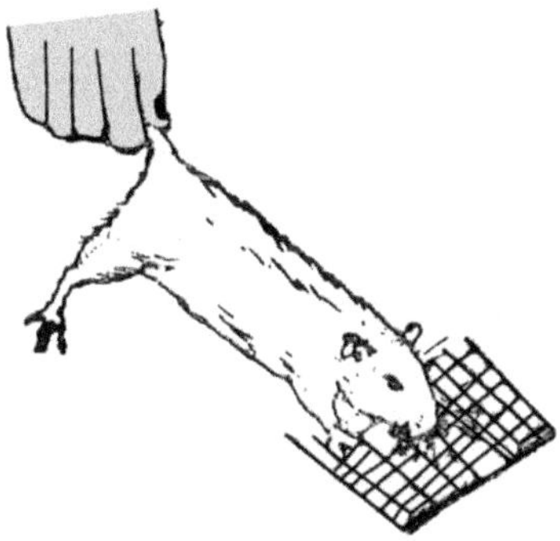

(a)

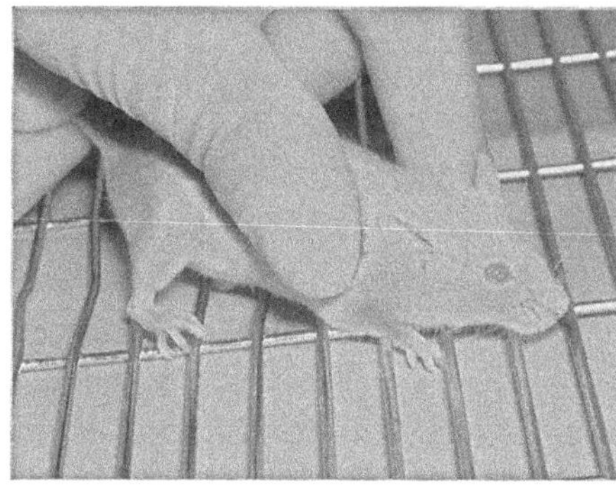

(b)

Fig. 1 Holding of Mouse, a, b.

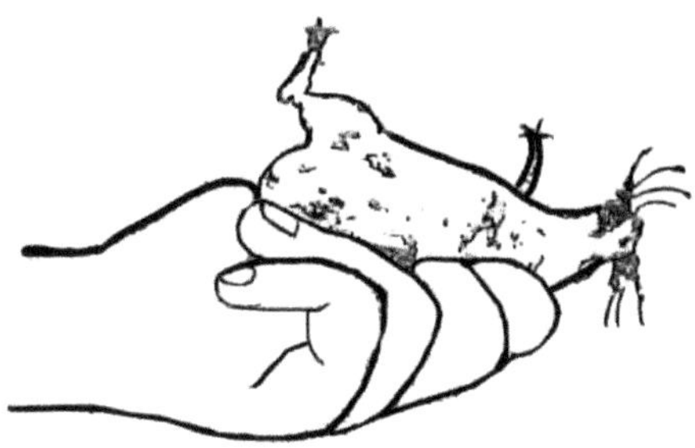

(c)

Fig. 1 Holding of Mouse, c.

Breeding of Mouse

The mouse is a prolific (fertile) breeder. Puberty occurs at the age of four to six weeks. However, mating is done when the animals are around 45-60 days old. Mice bred too early (less than six weeks of age) or too late (after ten weeks of age) causes reduction of fertility. 60 days old male mouse weighs around 35 gms. and the female around 30 gms.

Age at sexual maturity (days)	Breeding season	Estrus		Gestation Period (days)	Young No. / Litter
		Type	Cycle (days)		
30–45	all year	P	4	19–21	6-12

Inbred Strains of Mouse

A strain is considered as inbred when it has been mated full brothers and sisters (bxs) for 20 or more consecutive generations. Even then it is not completely inbred in the true sense because it gives an inbreeding co-efficient of only 98.6% which means that on the average 1.4% of the originally heterogygous genes are still heterogygous. The total list of inbred starins and clearly defined substrain now exceeds 300. Wide use of inbred strains has been found in almost every field of biomedical research. The chief drawbacks of inbred strain are that the animal become generally less healthy, more susceptible to disease and reproductive capacity is reduced (inbreeding depression).

Estrus Cycle of Mouse

The mouse is habituated to a recurring estrus cycle of four days' duration. At the interval of 4 days, the females being housed in close association with males, cycle regularly; and this is caused by a pheromone released by the males. Single female housed away from the males do not cycle regularly, or the interval between cycles tends to be longer in them. In case of large groups of females being housed together, they tend to go into anestrus and do not cycle, as because the females become pseudo, regnant and this is known as the "Lee-Bool-effect". Such group of females when accommodated with a male, begin to cycle, and come into estrus or heat, after about 72 hours exposure to the male. This phase is known as the "Whitten effect".

According to the cell types found in the vaginal smear, it is estimated that estrus cycle of the mouse is divided into five stages, viz pro-estrus, estrus (early), estrus (late), metestrus and diestrus. Being influenced by 'heat' or estrus, the female is most receptive to a male and mating will take place if a male is present with her in the same cage. But estrus cycle does not take place when the mouse is pregnant or lactating. However, immediately after delivery, the female leans to estrus and this stage of estrus is known as the post-partum estrus. Irregularity of estrus cycle occurs in the case of pseudopregnancy.

Mating Technique of Mouse

The monogamous and polygamous methods are resorted to usually. In the former system a male and a female are paired together and the youngs are segregated from the mother prior to the next parturition (act of bringing forth). By dint of this system the advantage of post-partum estrus is utilised to produce maximum number of litters within shortest time. For the purpose of evaluation of the individual female production, accurate breeding records have to be maintained. This system, however, creates disadvantages also. A good number of males have to be maintained in cages, which would entail increase of labour, enlargement of space and larger provision of equipments.

One male mouse is caged with 2 to 6 females while applying polygamous or harem method. Females with pregnancy are housed in a separate cage being removed from the group. After the weaning of young, the female is arranged to associate with a male for subsequent mating. By this system more youngs are weaned per litter and they are healthier than those raised by post partum matings, The total number of litters produced per breeder is fat less. Successful mating in mice can be determined by the detection of sperms in the vaginal smear or by the presence of a copulatory plug (solidified semen) in the vagina. The mouse introduced for mating should be examined everyday morning for the presence of copulatory plug. Pregnancy can be detected 'by palpating the animal around 8-10 days of gestation. Daily weighing will also reveal an increased rate of weight gain by about 13 days of gestation.

On an average, length of gestation extends to 19-21 days, but this may, however, prolong to 24 to 30 days in case of post-partum matings, according to the size of the suckling litter.

Timed Pregnancies of Mouse

Numerous ways of timed pregnancies in mice are noticed. Taking advantages of the rebound cycles that occur in the whitten effect is one way. And the other is to perform vaginal smears and mate only those mice in heat, which is however, time consuming. For the presence of vaginal plugs, mice has to be examined daily,

The size of litter differs considerably according to strain and age. The mouse gives birth to 6-12 pups per litter, the first litter being generally smaller. Till the age of about one year mice breed well and during this period 8 to 10 litters emerge per breeding. The productivity diminishes after the first 6 litters. The litters are likely to be comparatively less frequent and smaller in size and pre-weaning mortality is greater.

A new born (1 day old) pup weighs about one gm. Just at the point of birth the young are hairless and their eyes and ears remain completely closed. Hair on the body begins to grow after about 3 days of birth and within about 10 days hair coat fully covered; the eyes and ears open on attaining the age of 12-13 days. Pups attaining the age of 14-16 days start to eat solid food and they are weaned (separated from the mother) when they are 21 days old. At this age, weight around 10-14 gms. is noticed in each young.

Sexing of Mouse

One day-old mice even can be sexed by measuring the anogenital distance. This distance in male is greater than the same in female.

Life Span of Mouse

The longivity of laboratory mouse ranges from $1\frac{1}{2}$ years to $2\frac{1}{2}$ years.

Common Diseases of Mouse

Any element of extra stress on the animals metabolism may create to predispose them to disease. Poor or low nutrition, over-crossing, lack of hygiene, insufficient ventilation, rough handling and exposure (directly or by indirect contact) to mice suffering from infectious disease will all lead to an out break of disease in a colony.

A healthy mouse will be active with smooth and glossy coat. An ill mouse will be inactive and will have a rough haircoat. It will have no eagerness for food and will lose weight. Symptoms like conjunctivities, diarrhoea, accelerated respiration, wheezing or chattering, swelling on the tail, enlargement of feet, etc. are indicative of existence of some disease in mice.

Mice are sensitive to both streptomycin and chloroform. Mice often die if streptomycin is injected even in low concentrations. Many inbred strains of mice, particularly the males, are sensitive to chloroform vapour and may die following accidental exposure,

Collection of Blood from Mouse

Blood samples can be obtained from mice by cardiac puncture or tail vein puncture by needle (25 to 27 gauge and $\frac{1''}{2}$ to 1" long fitted with 1 or 2 ml syringe).

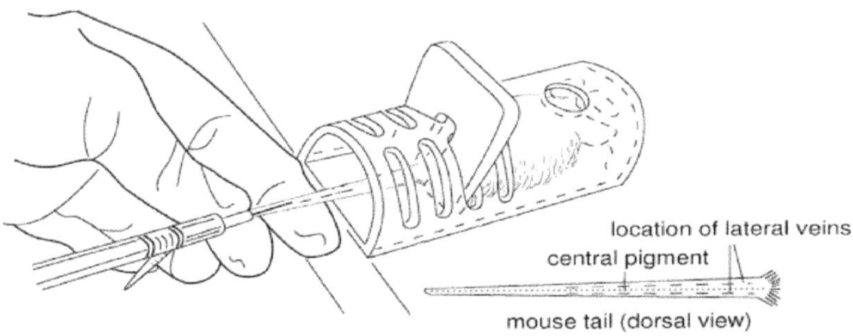

Fig. 2 Intravenous injection (Mice).

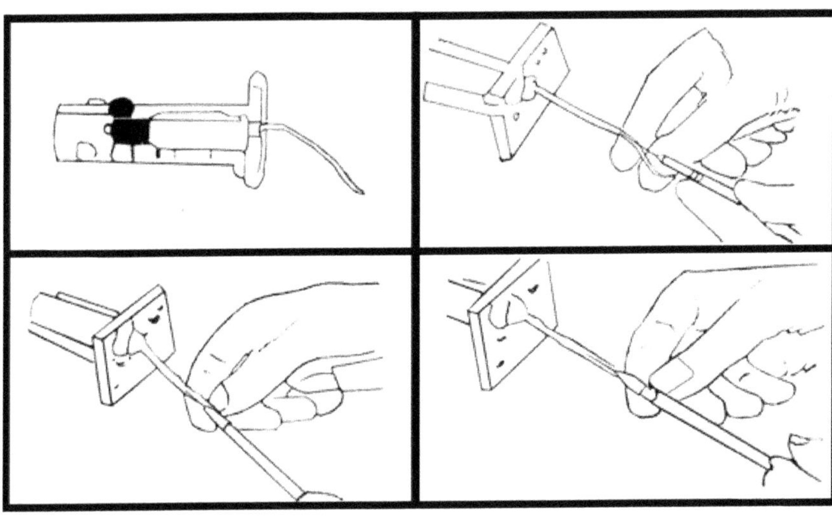

Fig. 3 Blood sample collection from mouse tail vein.

The most efficient method of collecting blood causing least strains to the animals is from orbital sinus with the help of a capillary tube. The animal is restrained in such a way that the loose skin of the head is tightened while holding the head with the left hand with the help of index finger when the eye is made to protrude by traction on the skin adjacent to the eye. The thumb is pressed just behind the angle of the jaw resulting in the engorgement of the retro orbital plexus. The tip of a blood pipette is then inserted at the medial canthus into retro orbital plexus with gentle rotation by the end of the other hand. As the vessels are ruptured, blood wells up in the periorbital space. The tip of the pipette is then slightly withdrawn so that the blood flows into the pipette by capillary action.

Bleeding stops once the normal ocular pressure is allowed to impinge on the venous plexus by releasing the animal.

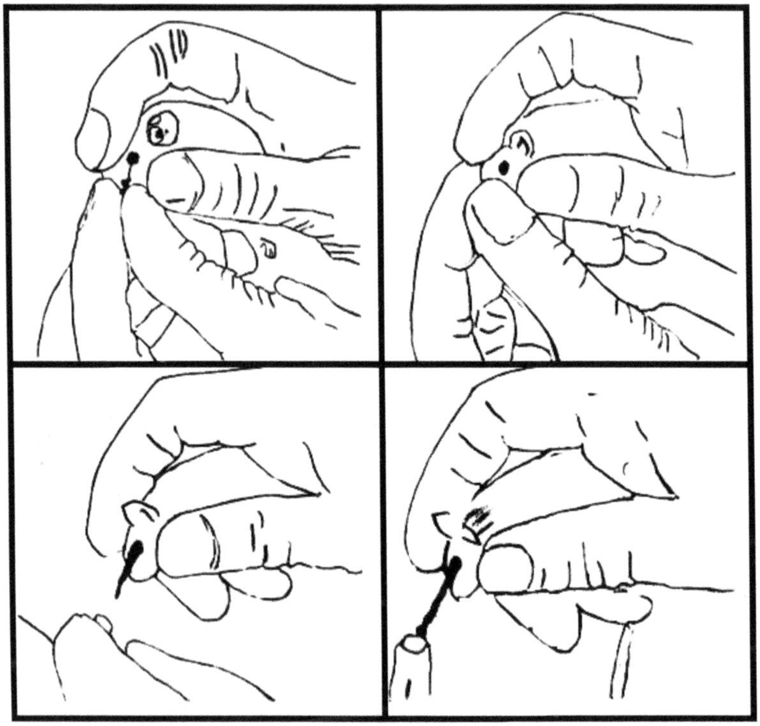

Fig. 4 Blood sample collection from mouse orbital sinus.

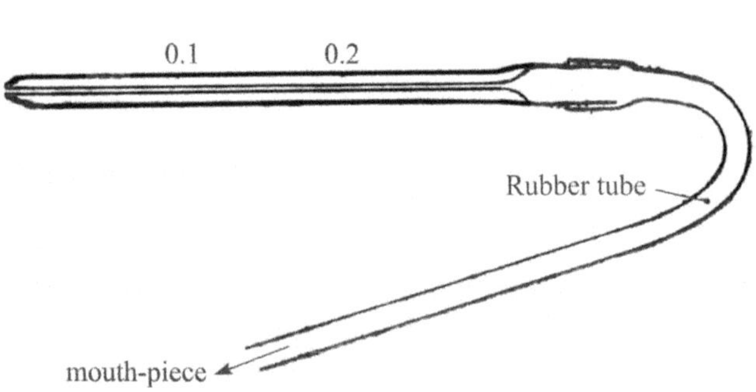

Fig. 5 A blood pipette.

The total volume of blood of a mouse is about 6- 8% of its body weight. A maximum of 7.7 ml. can be collected safely in one spell of bleeding.

Administration of Drug to Mouse

Administration of medications can be made by oral (p. o), subcutaneous (s. c), intramuscular (i. m), intraperitoneal (i. p) and intervenous (i. v) routes. Appropriate volume for injection is 1 ml / 100 gms body weight. Subcutanous injections can be made into the scruff of the neck. Intramuscular injection is given into the hind leg, whereas intravenous injection is usually

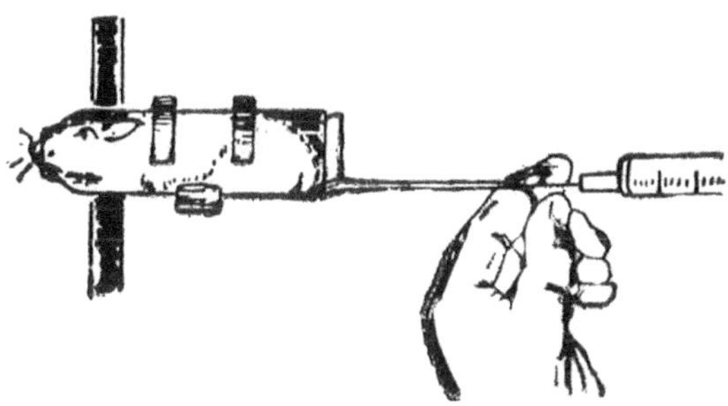

Fig. 6 I.V. injection to a mouse.

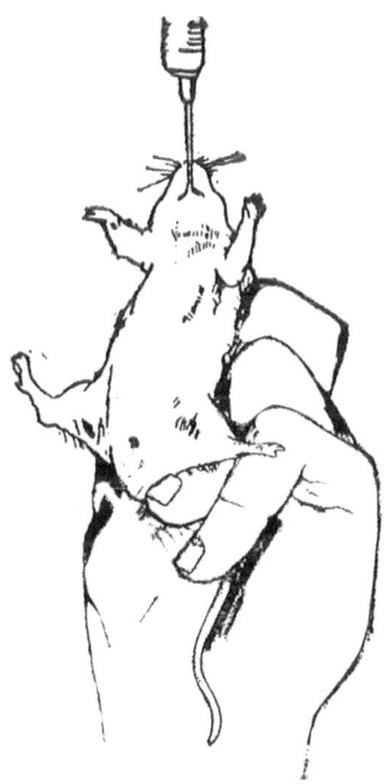

Fig. 7 P.O. injection to a mouse.

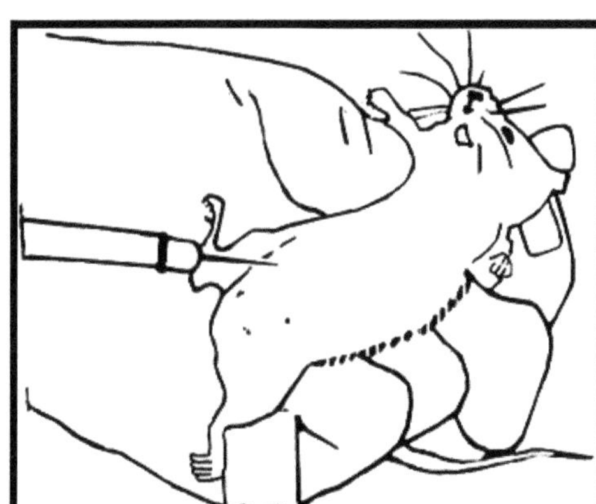

Fig. 8 P.O. injection to a mouse.

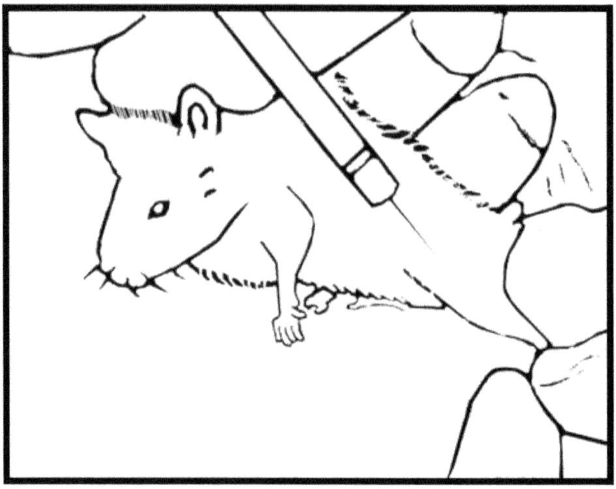

Fig. 9 Intramuscular injection (Mice)

given into the tail veins. The tail can be heated by dipping the same in warm water or rubbing it with xylene will make the tail vein to dilate becoming clearly visible, Intraperitoneal injections should be administered into lower, half of the abdomen on either side of the midline with the needle at about 1-20 degree angle to the skin.

Euthanasia of Mouse

Ether or carbondioxide in a jar can be used to kill mouse painlessly. Alternatively, the animal can be killed by cervical dislocation.

▲ Based on LAIS centre news.

DATA RELATED TO MICE

(Tables)

Table 1 Some Physiological Data of Mouse

Mature weight (gms.) Male/Female	Birth Weight (gms.)	Weaning Weight (gms.)	Weaning age (days)	Sexual Maturity age (days)	First Mating age (days)	Eyes open (days)	Begin eating solid food (days)	Litter size (av. No.)	Respiration rate/min. min. – mix.)
20-40 20-35	1.0-1.5	10-14	21	30-45	45-60	12-13	14-16	9	84-230

Table 2 Milk Composition of Mouse

Water (%)	Fat (%)	Protein(%)	Sugar (%)
75	10-12	9-11	3

Based on LAIS Centre News.

Table 3 Blood Pressure of Mouse

Systolic (mm. Hg)	Diastolic (mm. Hg)
113	81

Table 4 Heart Rate of Mouse

Specification body weight (gms)	Beats / min
Adult, Normal	(600-655)
10-20 gms. 38.4°C; awake	624 (480-738)
17 gms anaesthetized	(450-550)
29 gms anaesthetized	376

Table 5 Oxygen Consumption of Mouse

Age	Body weight (gms.)	Temperature °C		O_2 Consumption ml/gm/hr	Devitaion (%)
		Body	Ambient		
Adult	35.7	–	32	1.59	+4.6

Table 6 Respiratory Frequency, Tidal Volume and Minute Volume of Mouse

Body Weight (kg)	Condition of animal	Respiratory Frequency breaths/min.	Tidal Volume (ml)	Minute Volume (1trs / min.)
0.02 (0.012-0.026)	Normal	163 (84-230)	0.15 (0.09-0.23)	0.024 (0.011-0.036)

Table 7 Dimensions of Lung Respiratory Zones of Mouse

Specification *	Value
Wt, (kg)	0.023 $\pm$ 0.002
VL, (ml)	0.74 $\pm$ 0.075
Sa, (m^2)	0.068 $\pm$ 0.009
Sc, (m^2)	0.059 $\pm$ 0.006

Table 7 *Contd...*

Specification *	Value
Vc, (ml)	0.084 ± 0.009
τ. (μm)	1.25 ± 0.08
τht, (μm)	0.32 ± 0.006
τhp, (μm)	0.11 ± 0.002
τtmin	0.15
DL_{max}	0.147 ± 0.015
Sc : Sa	0.87
Vc/Sa (ml/m^2)	1.23

*Values derived from electron-microscopic studies. Specification : W_t = body weight, VL = lung volume, Sa = alveolar surface, Sc = capillary surface, Vc = capillary volume, τ = mean thickness of alveolar. Capillary tissue barrier thickness, τtmin = minimal barrier thickness, τhp = barmonic mean thickness of plasma layer DL_{max} = maximal diffusion capacity of lung. Sc:Sa ratio of capillary to alveolar surface, Vc/Sa = capillary volume per alveolar surface.

Table 8 Erythrocyte and Hemoglobin Values of Mouse

Erythro-cyte count million/μl of blood	Erthro-cyte packed volume ml/100 ml of blood	Erythro-cyte volume (μ^3)	Haemoglobin concentration		Erythro-cyte Haemo-globin content (pg)	Erythro-cyte dimen-sions (μ)
			gms/ 100 ml of blood	gms/ 100 ml of RBC		
9.3 (7.7-12.5)	41.5	49 (48-51)	14.8 10-19	36 (33-39)	16 (15.5-16.5)	6.0

Table 9 Leukocyte Counts of Mouse

Leukocytes, Total thousand/ μl of blood	Neutrophils thousands/ μl of blood	Eosinophils thousands/ μl of blood	Basophils thousands/ μl of blood	Lympho-cytes thousands/ μl of blood	Monocytes thousands / μl of blood
8.0 (4.0-12.0)	2.0 (0.7-4.0) 25.5 (12-44)%	0.15 (0.05) 2(0-5)%	0.05 (0-0.1) 0.5 (0-1)%	5.5 (3.0-8.5) 68 (54-85)%	0.3 (0-1.3) 4(0-15)%

Note: % of total leukocytes.

Table 10 Blood Platelet Counts of Mouse

Age, Sex	Platelets thousands/μl	Method used for estimation
Male (100-299 da)	937	Direct method, phase microscopy
Female (100-299 da)	924	

Table 11 Blood Carbohydrate of Mouse

Age and conditions	Blood Component	Carbo-hydrate Estima-ted	Concentration mg/100ml	Method of carbohydrate Estimation.
A	B	C	D	E
1 wk old,	Whole blood	Glucose	91 ± 2	Glucose Oxidase
55-33 wk old, fed ab lib.	Whole blood	Glucose	116 ± 13	Ferriferrocyanide
34 wk old	Whole blood	Glucose	134 ± 6	Glucose oxidase
Adult, Normal (female)	Serum	Glucose	66.6 ± 6.4	O -Toluidine
Adult, fed ad lib. nonanaesthetized	Whole blood	Glucose	173.8 ± 5.9	Ferriferrocyanide
Adult fasted 24 hrs. non-anaesthetized	Whole blood	Glucose	108.9 ± 3.6	Ferriferrocyanide
Adult, fed ad lib. nembutal anaesthesia	Whole blood	Glucose	70.1 ± 3.5	Ferriferrocyanide

Table 12 Blood Electrolytes of Mouse

Body weight (gms.)	Blood Component	Chemical Constituent	Concentration
25-35	Serum	Calcium	8.17 ± 0.18/-9.00 ± 0.19/mg/100 ml
25-35	Serum	Calcium	8.26 ± 0.16/-10.12 ± 0.18/mg/100 ml
20-25	Plasma	Calcium Chloride Phosphorus Potassium Sodium	2.78 ± 0.4 meq/ltr. 107.55 ± 6.66 meq/1tr. 6.55 ± 1.61 mg/100 ml. 5.25 ± 1.31 meq/1tr. 134.18 ± 9.58 meq/1tr.

Table 13 Blood Non-protein Nitrogenous Substances of Mouse

Age	Blood Component	Constituent	Concentration (mg/100ml blood)
Adult	Plasma	*Amino acids:*	
		Alanine	5.87 (5.3-6.61)
		Arginine	0.97 (0.9-1.0)
		Glutamic acid	3.33 (2.9-3.6)
		Glycine	1.90 (1.7-2.3)
		Histidine	1.57 (1.4-1.7)
		Isoleucine	1.47 (1.2-2.0)
		Leucine	2.40 (2.2-2.8)
		Lysine	6.37 (5.7 7.0)
		Methionine	1.9 (1.7-2.2)
		Phenylalanine	2.4 (2.0-3.2)
		Proline	1.83 (1.6-2.1)
		Threonine	3.50 (3.0-3.9)
		Tryptophan	1.23 (1.1-1.4)
		Tyrosine	2.53 (2.4-2.7)
		Valine	4.30 (3.8-5.0)

Table 14 Monoamines of Brain Tissue of Mouse

GABA (μg/gm of brain tissue)	NA (μg/gm of brain tissue)	A (μg/gm of brain tissue)	DA (μg/gm of brain tissue)	5 HT (μg/gm of brain tissue)
0.20 ± 0.03	0.16 ± 0.02	0.09 + 0.01	0.36 +0.04	0.4 ± 00.03

Table 15 Liver Function Tests of Mouse

Cholesterol (mg/100 ml. blood)	Bilirubin conjugated (ml/100 ml. blood)	Bilirubin (Total) (mg/100 ml of blood)	SGO-T (Units/ ml. Serum)	SGP-T (Units/ ml. Serum)	ALK-Phos-phatase (Units/ ml. Serum)	Acid Phos-phatase (Units/ ml. Serum)
98 ± 5.83	0.60 ± 0.12	1.60 ± 0.20	55.1 ± 2.01	28 ± 0.62	600 ± 90.0	0.70 ± 0.04

Table 16 Excretion Products in Urine of Mouse

Properties/Constituents	Value (μg/kg body wt/day)
Nitrogenous substances Amino acid : Taurine	11890**
Pyrimidine derivative: Deoxycytidine	(125-625)
Miscellaneous 4-Amino.5-imidazole-carboxamide	260
Homovanillic acid	40

* *Urine specification* : Clear yellow, pH 6.0, 4-7 ml/day output.

** After fasting

Table 17 Typical Electroencephalograms of Mouse

Age	Experimental condition of animal	Frequency (Hz)	Amplitude (μV)	Remarks
Adult	Alert	20-34	50-100	–
	Relaxed asleep	3-5	200-300	–
	Alert	8-16	50-100	"Activated' sleep Cortical theta
	Relaxed –asleep	2-8	100-200	–

Table 18 Tolerance to Temperature Extremes of Mouse

Age/ Body Weight	Tem Measured	Tolerance limit			Survival	Comments
		Extreme	Temp. °C	Duration		
A	B	C			D	E
3.5-11 mo.	Air	Lower	(1.5-6.5)	24 hrs	All Survived	Cold room
Adult	Air	Upper	37	3 hrs	Major survived	

Table 18 *Contd...*

Age/ Body Weight	Tem Measured	Tolerance limit			Survival	Comments
		Extreme	Temp. °C	Duration		
A	B	C			D	E
		Lower	5.8	2 mo.	All survived	Cold room, with daily temp range of 7°C (mean)
			–35	0.4 hrs.	All dead	Controlled temp. room; wind, 2 ml/hr.
20-27 (gms.)	Air	Lower	–9	200 min.	A few survived	Acclimated to 30°C
			–17	200 min.	A few survived	Acclimated to 20°C
			–20	200 min.	All dead	Acclimated to 10°C
			–22	200 min	All dead	Acclimated to 0°C

Table 19 Nutritional Requirement of Mouse

Part I General

Age	Specification of animal	Body weight (kg)	Avg. Daily Gain/ (gms.)	Daily Feed (gms.)	Protein		DE/, K_{cal} ME, M_{cal}]
					Total (gms.)	Digestoble (gms.)	
21-da Weaning	Growth	0.009-0.010	5-13 / 14 da	N.S	N.S	N.S	N.S
Adult	Pregnancy & Lactation	N.S	N.S	N.S	N.S	N.S	400/100 gms diet

Requirements are based on air dry feed containing 90% dry matter.

Part 1I Minerals

Age	Specifc ation of animal	Body Wei- ght (kg)	Avg. Daily Gain (gms)	Cal- ciu m gms	Io- dine mg.	Magne- sium (gms.)	Phos- phorous (gms)	Sodium + Chlorin e (gms.)
Adult *	Growth	0.021 - 0.6/1 00 gms. diet	N.S	N.S	N.S	N.S	0.018- 0.5/100 gms.	0.018- 0.5/100 gms.

*Also required: iron, manganese, potassium and zinc

Part III Vitamins

Age	Speci- fication	Ribo- flavin (mg)	Niacin (mg)	B_0 (mg)	Panto- thanic acid (mg)	B_{12} (μg)	A (IU)	D (IU)
	** Growth	> 0.4	1.0	0.4	> 0.85	>0.5	> 50	15
+ Adult	** Pregnancy and Lactation	0.7	N.S	N.S	1.02	0.05	>50	N.S

** Per 100gms diet : + Also required thiamine, biotin, folic acid, choline and α-tocopherol.

N.S – not specified.

Table 20 Parasitism in Mouse

(A. External, Parasities)

Species (Distribution) A	Incidence in Laboratory B	Effect on Host C
	Acarina	
A	**B**	**C**
Myobia muscult (World wide)	Common	Dermatitis, alopecia, pruritus, self-inflicted trauma, secondary amyloidosis.
Myocoptes musculinus (World wide)	Common	Pruritus, erythema, traumatic dermatitis, alopecia.
Psorergatas simples (possibly world wide)	Common	Caseous nodules in skin, dermal cysts; some-times scabby dermatitis of ears.
Radfordia affinis (Worldwide)	Common	Effects unknown; probably dermatitis, alopecia, pruritus.
Trichoecius romboutsi (United States, Europe)	Unknown	Effects unknown
	Siphonaptera	
Leptopsylla segnis (Worldwide)	Rate	Acts as intermediate host for *Hymenolepts diminuta & H. nana.*
	Mullophaga & Anoplura	
Polyplux serrata (Worldwide)	Common in some colonies rare or absent in others.	Pruritus, anemia, Vector of Eperythrozoon coccoides.

Table 20 *Contd...*

(B. Internal Parasities)

Species (Distribution)	Incidence in Laboratory	Host (Localization)	Effects on Host
A	B	C	D
Nematoda			
Aspiculuris tetraptera (Worldwide)	Common	Cecum	Usually nonpathogenic heavy infections some times cause impaction, intussusceptions rectal prolapsed.
S. Obvelate (Worldwide)	Common	Cecum, colon	Usually nonpathogenic heavy infections some times cause impaction, intussuception, rectal prolapsed.
Platyhelminthes – Cestoda			
Hymenolepsis diminuta (Worldwide)	Uncommon	Intestine	Usually inapparent; sometimes enteritis.
H. nana (Worldwide)	Common	Intestine	Retarded growth, weight loss.
T. taeniaeformis (Worldwide)	Common in some colonies, absent in others	Liver	Hepatic cyst formation; sometimes hepatic sarcoma,
Protozoa			
E. falciformis (Worldwide)	Common in some colonies, absent in others	Intestine	Anorexia, diarrhea, catarrhal enteritis; sometimes death.
Hexamita Muris (Worldwide)	Common in some colonies, absent in others.	Small Intestine, cecum.	Associated with duodenitis.
K. muris (Worldwide)	Common in some colonies, absent in others	Kidneys	Usually none; sometimes necrotic foci in kidneys.
Nosema Cuniculi (Worldwide)	Common in some colonies, uncommon in others.	Brian, Kidneys, other tissue	Usually inapparent; sometimes encephalitis, nephritis, death.

Table 20 *Contd...*

A	B	C	D
Toxoplasma gondii (Worldwide)	Common in some colonies; uncommon or absent in others	Various tissues	Inapparent to fatal disease with varied signs.

(C. Viral Diseases)

Virus Group [Examples]	Morphology [Nucleic Acid]	Host [Natural Transmission]	Remarks
A	B	C	D
Coronaviruses mouse hepatitis; viruses causing acute upper respiratory infection	Pleomorphic 80-160 nm electron-trans-parent core; envelope with projections [RNA]	Respiratory; in feces	Hemagglutinins not demonstrated
Tacaribe-LCM viruses-Lymphocytic choriomeningitis; viruses causing South American hemorrhagic fevers.	Similar to toga viruses larger upto 110 nm [Single stranded [RNA]	Anthropod vectors, in feces & urine	Virion contains granules similar to ribosomes

(D. Rickettsial Parasites)

Species	Disease or Disorder	Method of Transmission
Haemobartonella SPP.	Haemobartonellosis, anemia	Flea to host
Rickettsia akari	Rickettsial pox	Mite to mouse
R. sibirica	Siberian tick typhus	Tick to host
R. tsutsugamushi	Tsutsugamushi fever (scrub typhus)	Mite to mouse
R. typhi	Murine or endemic typhus	Flea faces.
Ricolesia bovis	Infectious conjuctivitis	Contact

Table 21 Chemical Composition of Nervous Tissue of Mouse

Tissue Specification	Age	Chemical Constituent	Concentration
A	B	C	D
Nervous tissue	Adult	Allanine	0.66 μ mole/gm.
		β-Alanine	0.05 μ mole/gm
		Arginine	0.13 μ mole/gm
		Aspartic acid	3.4 μ mole/gm
		L. Cystathionine	0.06 μ mole/gm
		Cysteine	0.01 μ mole/gm
		Glutamic acid	12 μ mole/gm
		Glutamine	6.6 μ mole/gm
		Glycine	1.6 μ mole/gm
		Histidine	0.05 μ mole/gm
		Isoleucine	0.04 μ mole/gm
		Leucine	0.08 μ mole/gm
		Lysine	0.18 μ mole/gm
		Methionine	0.03 μ mole/gm
		Ornithine	0.01 μ mole/gm
		Phenylalanine	0.04 μ mole/gm
		Proline	0.06 μ mole/gm
		Serine	0.78 μ mole/gm
		Taurine	9.1 μ mole/gm
		Threonine	0.39 μ mole/gm
		Tyrosine	0.05 μ mole/gm
Nervous tissue	Adult	Sterol	41 mg/gm.
		Protein	190 mg/gm*
Sciatic nerve		H_2O	59% by wt.
		Cl	50 μ mole/gm
		K	57 μ mole/gm
		Na	78 μ mole/gm
Microsomes		Phosphatidal & phosphatidyl choline	103 mg/gm +
		Phospatidal Phosphatidyl Ethanolamine	123 mg/gm +
		Phosphatidal & phosphatidyal serine & Phosphatidyl inositals	68 mg/gm +

Table 21 *Contd...*

Tissue Specification	Age	Chemical Constituent	Concentration
A	B	C	D
		Sphingomyelin Cerebroside Sulfatide Cholesterol	52 mg/gm. + 55 mg/gm. + 5 mg/gm. + 162 mg/gm. +

* Estimated by difference of dry weight minus total lipids

\+ Dry weight.

Table 22 Tissue Growth And Renewal In Mouse

Organ	Growth specification	Age/other specification	Tissue growth & renewal
A	B	C	D
		Nervous System	
Brain & spinal cord	Proliferation	11-da embryo	Neuroepithelium: $T_c \approx 11$ hr ; $T_s \approx 5.5$ hr.
		15-da embryo	Neuroepithelium : $T_c \approx$ 11-12 hr ; $T_s \approx 7$ hr. cell
	Mode of growth	N. S.	Proliferation in embryonic development & growth; mainly cytoplasmic growth in postnatal development; DNA concentration decreased 380 mg/100 gms. Wet wt in subjects 1-2 da old, & 240 mg/100 gms. Wet wt in subjects 3-6 months old.
	Life span		Coextensive with normal function.
	Replacement		None in neurons; neuroglial cells renewed slowly.

Table 22 *Contd...*

Organ	Growth specification	Age/other specification	Tissue growth & renewal
A	B	C	D
	Regenerative capacity		In very young subjects, CNS outgrowth occurs from neuroblasts ; in adults, some axonal growth occurs after section; sprouting from intact central axons occurs in damaged region, but functional recovery is minimal. Neuroglia are capable of proliferation.
Cerebellum	Proliferation	3wk old	Proliferative external granular layer present from which basket cells are formed.
Digestive System			
Alimentary canal:Buccal mucosa	Proliferation	N. S.	T_c = 80-100 hr; T_s = 7-8 hr LI = 6-8% ; MI = 17-2.6%
Gingivae	Replacement	N. S.	Epithelium : T_t = 4-5 da
Lips	Replacement	N. S.	Epithelium : T_t = 7-8 da
Tongue	Proliferation	N. S.	Epithelium : T_c = 80-90 hr ; 21-35 hr ; LI of basal layer = 11-21% ; LI variation due to diurnal rhythm Mean MI of basal layer for 24-hr period = 6.6%
	Replacement	N. S.	Epithelium : T_t = 1-8 da
Esophagus	Proliferation	N. S.	T_c = 87 hr; T_m = 0.7 hr 34 T_s = 7 hr, LI = 1-11% MI = 0.8%
Digestive System			
Fore-stomach	Proliferation	N. S	T_c = 28-55 hr T_s = 7 hr ; LI = 3-14% ; marked diurnal rhythm & variation among animals.

Table 22 *Contd...*

Organ	Growth specification	Age/other specification	Tissue growth & renewal
A	B	C	D
	Life span	N. S.	Cells in basal layer ; 40 hr Cells in superficial layer: 55 hr
Duodenum	Proliferation	N. S.	T_c = 10-17 hr ; T_s = 7-11 hr, depending on age, strain, & flora, $T_m \approx 1$ hr. 15.2 cells/ crypt/hr are produced, and 855 crypts/mg wet wt are present.
	Proliferation	Weaning	MI = 3.4 %
		54 & 147 da old	T_c = 10-11 hr, T_s = 7 hr, Tm = 0.7-1 hr.
		Adult	MI = 5.6 %
	Mode of growth	17th da of gestation of birth	Absolute & relative weights of intestine increase.
		2-15 da old	Absolute weight of intestine increases slowly.
		23-48 da old	Absolute & relative weights of intestine increase, body & intestine weights increase at same rate.
	Life span & replacement	N. S.	T_t = 1.7-2-2 da, depending on age & strain
Jejunum	Proliferation	N. S.	T = 11-18 hr T_s = 7-8 hr. Proliferation shows diurnal fluctuation.
	Life span & replacement	N. S.	T_t = 2-3 da
Ileum	Proliferation	N. S.	T_c = 11-7 hr, T_s = 6-8 hr.
	Life span & replacement	N. S.	T_t = 1-3 da, longer in germ-free subjects.
Total small intestine	Regenerative capacity,	N. S.	Mucosal wounds are repaired at all levels by epithelial migration & proliferation.

Table 22 *Contd...*

Organ	Growth specification	Age/other specification	Tissue growth & renewal
A	B	C	D
Colon	Proliferation	Infant, adult, senescent	T_c = 15 hr, T_c = 16-19 hr, T_c = 21 hr, T_s = 7-9 hr.
	Regenerative capacity	N. S.	Mucosal repair and new gland formation occur; variations are due to amount of granulation.
Parotid	Proliferation	N. S.	LI = 0.07-0.50% increases to ≈ 22%, 25 hr after isoproterenol is given.
Liver	Proliferation	N. S.	T_s = 7-8 hr. LI = 0.02-0.53% Littoral cells : LI = 1.2-1.5%; increases to 7-22% with estradiol or zymosan.
	Regenerative capacity	N. S.	Can occur repeatedly, Normal weight almost regained 8 da after two-thirds hepatectomy. Age affects regenerative capacity.
Pancreas	Proliferation	Embryo	Beta and exocrine gland clles ; T_c = 32-91 hr. Beta aciner, and duct cells; T_s ≈ 6 hr. Islet and exocrine gland cells; LI = 0.8 %.
		14 da	Differentiated beta cells appear.
		15 da adult	DNA synthesis detected. Acinar cells : T_s ≈ 8 hr.
Circulatory System			
Heart	Mode of growth	2 da old	Muscle cells : LI 4 hr after labeling = 8.3%
		3 wk old	Muscle cells : LI 4 hr after labeling = 0.15 %.
		Adult	No proliferative cells seen in muscle.

Table 22 *Contd...*

Organ	Growth specification	Age/other specification	Tissue growth & renewal
A	**B**	**C**	**D**
	Replacement	N. S.	No
	Regenerative capacity	N. S.	Probably negligible, hypertrophy caused by increased fiber size,
Endocardium	Proliferation	N. S.	LI = 1.9%
Epicardium	Proliferation	N. S.	LI = 0.7 %
Blood : Erythrocytes and precursors	Proliferation	N. S.	T_c = 3.5 hr; T_s = 4.5 hr ; T_m = 0.2 hr. LI = 19% MI ≈ 2.0%
	Life span	N. S.	20-45 da
Lymphocytes	Proliferation	N. S.	T_c = 8-13 hr. T_s = 5-hr, T_m = 0.5 hr, LI = 39% on 3rd day of primary response. In thymus ; T_c = 6.8-2.2 hr ; T_S = 5.5 hr ; TG1 = 1.4 hr ; In spleen germinal centres ; T_c = 13.4 hr. Ts = 4.5 hr. LI = 19.2%. In mesenteric lymph nodes LI = 22.3%. precursors to antibody-forming cells. Peak LI = 4-6.5 % on 6th day of secondary response,
	Life span	N. S.	Wide variation in life spans. Some survive > 1 yr. Bone marrow lymphocytes are probably short-lived, and ≈ one third of the blood lymphocytes are short-lived Long-lived lymphocytes recirculate from lymph to blood, and have potential for division and immunological competence.

Table 22 *Contd...*

Organ	Growth specification	Age/other specification	Tissue growth & renewal
A	B	C	D
	Replacement	N. S.	Thoracic duct : (30-60) × 10^6 cells/hr , Thymus : $T_t \approx$ 60 hr. Thymus can produce no, equal to total lymphocytes in body in 2-3 da
Platelets	Production	N. S.	Maturation occurs from stem cell- Poly ploid precursor cell. megakaryo-blast (stage I) promega-karyocyte (stage II) platelets are then formed by fragmentation of granular megakaryocyte cytoplasm (Stage-III)
		N. S.	Stages I and II take 50-57 hr.
	Life span	N. S.	4 da
Lymphatic System			
Thymus	Proliferation	N. S.	Mitosis in PAS ± Positive/ reticulum cells and medullary epithelial cells of adults. MI highest in neonatal period; higher in female, and varies with strain. Asymmetrical divisions sustain ratio of lymphocyte; T_c = 6-8 hr, T_S = 5.5 hr. MI = 1% medium lymphocytes: T_s = 8.2 hr. MI = 10%. Small lymphocytes; LI ≈ 2; most are nondividing cells.
	Mode of growth	N. S.	Atrophy in old age affects cortex more than medulla.

Table 22 *Contd...*

Organ	Growth specification	Age/other specification	Tissue growth & renewal
A	B	C	D
	Replacement	N. S.	Primitive thymic cells are continuously replaced by blood-borne lymphocytes. Total population is replaced every 3-4 da; most cells produced in thymus die *in situ*, <5% thymic lymphocytes may have a longer intrathymic life span.
+ PAS = periodic acid-schiff reaction.			
Urogenital System			
Kidney	Proliferation	N. S.	Tubular epithelium : $T_s = 7$ hr ; LI = 0.4-1.2%, MI is inversely related to function
Bladder	Proliferation	N. S.	Transitional epithelium : LI = 0.1-2.1 % ; MI = 0.01%.
Bladder & ureter	Regenerative capacity	N. S.	Regeneration of transitional epithelium by division of basal layer and superficial hyperdiploid cells.
Testis	Duration of spermatogenesis	N. S.	26-35 da; average length of supermatogenic wave = 12-30 mm.
Spermafogonia	Regenerative capacity	N. S.	Regeneration after injury occurs if spermatogonia type A survive.
Type AII	Proliferation	N. S.	$T_c = 27\text{-}31$ hr ; $T_s = 6$ hr ; LI = 20%
Type AIII	Proliferation	N. S.	$T_c = 27\text{-}31$ hr ; $T_s = 8$ hr ; LI = 29%
Type AIV	Proliferation	N. S.	$T_c = 27\text{-}31$ hr ; $T_S = 12$ hr ; LI = 40%

Table 22 *Contd...*

Organ	Growth specification	Age/other specification	Tissue growth & renewal
A	B	C	D
Intermediate	Proliferation	N. S.	T_c = 27-31 hr ; T_s = 13 hr ; LI = 46%.
Type B	Proliferation	N. S.	T_c = 30 hr ; $T_s \approx$ 15 hr ; LI = 49%
Spermato-cytes	Proliferation	N. S.	T_s = 14 hr.
Spermatozoa	Life span	N. S.	13.5 hr
Ovary	Regenerative capacity	N. S.	Compensatory hypertrophy after unilateraloophorecto-may or partial resection and hormonal stimulation
Medium sized	Proliferation	21 da old	T_S = 9.8-11.2 hr ; LI = 8.5-17.3% Granulosa cells : doubling time = 46-84 hr.
		28 da old	LI = 9.5-17.1%
		35 da old	LI = 8.3-16.4% Granulosa cells: doubling time = 46-76 hr.
Large sized	Proliferation	21 da old	T_s = 6.8 hr ; LI = 30-31% Granulosa cells : doubling time = 9 hr.
		28 da old	LI = 35-38.7%
		35 da old	LI = 32.6-35.4% Granulosa cells : Doubling time = 15.4-17.0 hr.
Graafian	Proliferation	N. S.	Granulosa cells proliferate.
Oocytes	Proliferation	N. S.	Occurs in fetal period.
	Regenerative capacity	N. S.	No regeneration
Uterus Bndometrium	Proliferation & mode of growth	Metestrus, 2 hr	Surface epithelium : LI = 60%. Glandular epithelium LI = 40%.Connective tissue LI= 0.62%

Table 22 *Contd...*

Organ	Growth specification	Age/other specification	Tissue growth & renewal
A	B	C	D
		Pregnant	Deciduomata : Formed decidual cells complete proliferation by time of implantation by time of implantation but decidual cell population increases by migration from adjacent areas
		2nd da	LI decreases.
		3rd -6th da	LI<5%
		4th da	Proliferative activity varies in relation to proximity to implantation area.
		5th da	Stromal cells: LI = 55.4%
		5th-6th da	Decidual cells : T_c = 10-11hr ; T_s < 5 hr ; TG2 = 1-2.5 hr; TG_1 + T_m = 3.5-4 hr.
		After estrogen	T_c = 26 hr ; T_s = 5.5 hr. Surface epithelium ; LI = 7.0 % Glandular epithelium LI = 4.0%
		Castrate	$T_c \approx$ 42 hr ; T_s = 8.5 hr. Surface epithelium : LI = 3.0% ; MI = 0.23% Glandular epithelium : LI = 5.0% ; MI = 0.4%
Vagina	Proliferation	Early diestrus	LI = 5.7-8.1%
		Diestrus	T_c = 72 hr; T_S = 7-5 hr ; LI = 10.4%
		Mid-to late diestrus	LI = 13.5-18.8%
		Proestrus	LI = 32.9%
		Estrus	T_c = hr ; T_s = 7.6 hr ; LI = 25.3-34.6%
		Late estrus	LI = 9.2-12.8% ;

Table 22 *Contd...*

Organ	Growth specification	Age/other specification	Tissue growth & renewal
A	B	C	D
		After esterogen	Newly formed cells in basal layer differentiate.
		After progesterone	Basal cell proliferation accelerates.
		Castrate 12 hr after estrogen	Basal layer : LI rises from 3% to 40%.
		24 hr after estrogen	Basal layer : MI rises from 0.01% to 2.4%.
	Replacement	N. S.	Cells produced in a basal layer move to vaginal lumen surface by end of estrus cycle.
Smooth muscle	Regenerative capacity	N. S.	Limited : regeneration after injury ; fibrous scar usual. In gut, hypertrophy and some proliferative activity occur.
Striated muscle	Mode of growth	N. S.	Cell division development.
		Adult	Hypertrophy
	Replacement	N. S.	Little or none.
	Regenerative capacity	N. S.	Restricted regeneration by satelite cells which divide and function as syoblasts.
Integumentary System			
Skin	Proliferation	N. S.	T_c = 4.2-6.5 da T_s = 5-8 hr/LI = 0.5 hr.
		New born	MI = 2-4%
		Hairless	T_c = 3-5 da T_s = 5-7 hr.
	Replacement	N. S.	Adjustment between cell loss and cell formation. Differentiated cells remain in basal layer 60 hr before moving to superficial layer.
		Hairless	Differentiated cells remain in basal layer ≈ 60 hr before moving to superficial layers.

Table 22 *Contd...*

Organ	Growth specification	Age/other specification	Tissue growth & renewal
A	B	C	D
	Regenerative capacity	N. S.	Re-epithelialization of wounds by proliferation and migration of cells ; amount of proliferation depends on size of wound. Regeneration possible from hair follicles. Growth granulation tissue checked by epithelium overgrowth.
Epidemis			T_c = 30-100 hr T_s = 18-30 hr
Ear	Proliferation	N. S.	LI = 2-3.8 hr
Skin out-growths :	Proliferation	N. S.	Follicle cells T_c = 11-13 hours, T_s = 1-8.5 hours
Hair	Hair cycle	N. S.	Waves of hair growth sweep prosteriorly and dorsally ; become less frequent with age. Follicle growth phase = 17-19 da
Nails	Growth rate	22-734 da old	0.01-0.126 cm/da
Endocrine Glands			
Para-thyroid gland	Proliferation	8 da old 18 da old 28 da old	MI = 0.07 % MI = 0.71 % MI = 0.01 %
Cortex	Proliferation	N. S.	Inner portion : T_s = 7.5, LI = 0.4-0.8 %
Medulla	Proliferation	N. S.	LI = 0.2-0.7 %
Thyroid gland	Proliferation	N. S.	LI = 0.6 %

* **Tissue Growth & Renewal Characteristics :** T_c = duration of cycle ; T_m = duration of mitosis, TG_1 = duration of pre-DNA synthesis ; T_s = duration of DNA synthesis phase ; TG_2 = duration of post-DNA synthesis ; T_t = turnover time (time taken to produce a number of cells equivalent to the total population studied) : LI : labeling index, measured in % cells in DNA synthesis ; MI = mitotic index, measured in % cells in mitosis. (if labeling and mitotic indexes are to be used in calculations, it must be known whether the index is based on total cell population, or on only the proliferative cells of a tissue).

N. S. = Not specified

Table 23 Inbred Strains of Mouse

Sl. No	Strain identification	Generations	Characteristics of inbred strain
A	B	C	D
1.	A	130	Low incidence of lung tumors and leukemia ; high incidence of mammary cancer in breeders, low in virgins, sporadic incidence of cleft palate, easily induced by a variety of agents high incidence of amyloidosis, renal disease in older animals.
2.	A/He	150	Same as strain A
3.	A/J	148	Same as strain A but lower percentage of granulocytes than in other strain A sublines
4.	A/Sn	N. A	25 presacral (7 cervical, 13 thoracic, 5 lumbar) vertebrae, high level of lipid in suprarenal glands, useful in transplantation studies.
5.	AKR	101	Incidence of leukemia 80-100% in some sublines, blood catalase activity high, a subline is sourse of suprarenalcortical lipid-depletion gene.
6.	AL/N	148	Very low incidence of mammary tumors, good fertility.
7.	AU	34	Do not reject (female) isografts (male)
8.	BALB/C	144	Low incidence of mammary tumors (susceptible of mammary tumor agent), and of leukemia, moderate incidence of lung tumors, some ovarian and suprarenal tumors, extremely sensitive to radiation, blood pressure heighest of 8 strains tested some heart lesions in old breeders, arteriosclerosis common, relatively nonaggressive.
9.	BALB/cCd	34	60-70 % of develop spontaneous bilateral adenocarcinoma of the kidney at 9-15 mo.
10.	BALB/Gw	75	Low resistance to Salmonelia typhimurium, same gynandromorphs.

Table 23 *Contd...*

Sl. No	Strain identification	Generations	Characteristics of inbred strain
A	B	C	D
11.	BC	60	Low incidence of mammary tumor and lymphoma, susceptible to X-ray or estrogen induction of lymphomas, estrogen treatment of hyphophyseal tumors, very few mammary rudiments in, high incidence of imperforate vagina, early genital atrophy in female.
12.		76	Resistant to *Salmonella*, some encephalitic viruses, and experimental allergic encephalomyelitis, thymus larger than that is BSVS strain and increases more under entigenic stimulation.
13.	BSVS	88	Susceptible to *Salmonella,* some encephalitic viruses, & experimental allergic encephalomyelitis.
14.	BT	35	Cortisone cause high fetal death rate, but low incidence of cleft palate in survivors.
15.	C	116	Moderate incidence of mammary tumors.
16.	CBA/ca	68	Some mammary tumors in breeders ; few skeletal variants ; ≈ 18% lack lower 3rd molars.
17.	CBA/J	149	Incidence of mammary tumors, 60%-65% in breeders, incidence of hepatomas, 65% in male; susceptible to whole-body irradiation; cleft palate induced by cortisone in ≈ 12% of strain
18.	CBA/H-T6	38	Homozygous for cytologic marker translocation T 6.
19.	CE	56	Low incidence of mammary tumors ; incidence of ovarian tumors, 33% after 20 mo ; high incidence of suprarenalcortical carcinoma in male/female after neonatal gonadectomy ; many tumor types ; high level of lipid in suprarenal glands.

Table 23 *Contd...*

Sl. No	Strain identification	Generations	Characteristics of inbred strain
A	B	C	D
20.	C3H	128	Incidence of mammary tumors up to 100% in breeding female, 85% in virgins ; hepatomas in male ; cleft palate induced by cortisone in 70% of strain ; low erythrocyte & leukocyte counts ; high mortality in male exposed to turpentine or chloroform fumes; calcareous heart deposits in most retired breeders.
21.	C2Hf	86	Low incidence of mammary tumors male have some hepatomas,
22	C57BL/Ks	77	High incidence of toe malformations ; microphthaimia ; high incidence of transient alopecia control for diabetic mutation (db) which across in this strain.
23.	C57BL/6	104	Low or no incidence of mammary tumors ; high incidence of hepatomas after irradiation ; incidence of eye defects, ≈ 12 % ; resistant to radiation ; cleft palate induced by cortisone in 20% of strain ; blood pressure range medium, high incidence of preference for alcohol, low level of lipid in suprarenal glands, high incidence of skeletal malformations
24.	C57BL/10	108	Occasional veginal septa, skeletal malformations.
25.	C57BR/cd	140	Low incidence of mammary tumors, incidence of hepatomas, 25% in male, very resistant to X-radiation, very sensitive to insulin.
26.	C57BR/z	>49	Low incidence of mammary tumors.
27.	C57L	116	Low, incidence of mammary tumors, some hypophyseal tumors in old animals ; hematocrit extremely high ; congenital cystic ovaries frequent.
28.	C58	150	Incidence of lymphatic leukemia 75%-95% in male & female, fairly low incidence of mammary tumors in virgins, higher in breeders, frequent polyvular follicles, ≈ 10% incidence of aplasia of the kidney.

Table 23 *Contd...*

Sl. No	Strain identification	Generations	Characteristics of inbred strain
A	B	C	D
29.	DBA/I	75	Resistant to most DBA/2 strain incidence of varied tumors at autopsy 22%, high incidence of mammary tumors in some sublines, cleft palate induced by cortisone in 90% of strain, high erythrocyte count, calcareous heart deposits in almost all retired breeders.
30.	DBA/2	105	Resistant to most DBA/1 strain tumors (P 1534 grows in 50% of strain, S91 grows in both strains), widely variable incidence of mammary tumor among substrains low incidence of leukemia, incidence of audiogenic seizures, 100% at 35 da, 5% after 55 da, high mortality in exposed to chloroform fumes, low blood pressure & low preference for alcohol, high erythrocyte count, low level of lipid in suprarenal glands, calcareous heart deposits in old animals.
31.	DBA/2 eB	35	Low incidence of mammary tumors, incidence of type B reticulum cells, 7.6% in virgins, 17.6% in breeders.
32.	DBAf	41	Lacks mammary tumor agent-no or low incidence of mammary tumors.
33.	DD	50	Incidence of mammary tumors 75% in virgins, 84% in breeders (some tumors arising in plaques).
34.	DE	61	High incidence of amyloidosis, polydipsia (30-50 ml da) and polyuria (25-45 ml da) more noticeable in female, no hypophyseal lesions, but kidneys & suprarenal glands are affected.
35.	DW	43	Dwarf, useful for endocrine studies
36.	F	113	High incidence of leukemia in older animals regardless of breeding conditions or sex.
37.	GR/A	50	In breeding female, high incidence of mammary tumors which are highly responsive to hormones, mammary tumor agent present, but not dependent on milk transmission.

Table 23 *Contd...*

Sl. No	Strain identification	Generations	Characteristics of inbred strain
A	B	C	D
38.	HRS/J	45	Incidence of leukemia in hairless mice, 45% at 8-10 mo. 72% at 18 mo, in haired controls, 1% at 10 mo, 20% at 18 mo. Useful for skin testing of chemicals.
39.	I	95	Resistant to chemical carcinogenesis, sex-linked phosphorylase kinase deficiency. Useful for nutrition studies.
40.	IF	91	No spontaneous mammary tumors, but high sensitivity to mammary tumor agent or to chemical induction, susceptible to ovarian tumor induction by chemicals, high incidence of spontaneous pseudopreganancy.
41.	KE	59	Low percentage of ova fertilized 17.6% of sperm have abnormal heads, mean litter size, 6.
42.	KK	57	Frequent diabetes mellitus (apparently not a unit character) occasional obesity in old mice, especially in the presence of the yellow gene, poor reproduction.
43.	KP	58	High embryonal & postembroynal mortality, low sperm production, abnormalities of tests.
44.	LG	51	≈ 10% incidence of lymphatic leukemia, body wt, 1.8 g at birth, 20.1 g at 28 da, 37.4 g at 60 da, not overly inclined to obesity, docile, low thyroid activity.
45.	LP	87	Incidence of varying types of late occurring tumors, 19% in male, 55% in female, mean life span, 750 da in male, 800 da in virgin female, high level of lipid in suprarenal glands in both.
46.	MA	90	Incidence of gross tumor 0% in male 5% in female, low incidence of mammary tumors, incidence of polydipsia-polyuria, 12% in male 79% in virgin female, incidence of gross kidney disease, 25% in male, incidence of hypophyseal cysts, 50%, high resistance to chronic whole-body X-irradiation.

Table 23 *Contd...*

Sl. No	Strain identification	Generations	Characteristics of inbred strain
A	B	C	D
47.	N	100	Low incidence of tumors, resistant to chemical carcinogenesis.
48.	NH	70	Low incidence of tumors, nodular hyperplasia & suprarenal adenomas in 10% of old mice (gonadectomy at 8 wk enhances adenomas)
49.	NZB/B1	86	Auto-immune hemolytic anemia extra-medullary erythropoiesis, glomerular & tubular renal lesions.
50.	NZBR/BI	---	Brown coat.
51.	NZC/BI	96	Low incidence of mammary cancer, increasing incidence of adenoacanthoma, congenital cystic kidney anomaly.
52.	NZO/BI	88	Low incidence of mammary tumor, high incidence of lung adenoma ; benign tumors of small intestine, obese.
53.	NZX/BI	52	Some incidence of imperforate vegina, low incidence of megacolon.
54.	NZY/BI	92	High incidence of mammary cancer associated with enlargement of hypophysis in breeding female, heritable megacolon.
55.	020	160	Very low incidence of mammary tumors, susceptibility to mammary tumor tumor agent which can be transmitted to offspring.
56.	P/J	110	Fairly low incidence of tumors, high resistance to chronic whole body X-irradiation, some polycystic or granular kidneys in both sex.
57.	PBA	42	Incidence of lymphomas, 100% at 35 wk, incidence of mammary tumors, 75% at 38 wk in breeding female, incidence of pulmonary adenomas, 77 % by 1 yr.
58.	PET	64	Occasional mammary tumors in old, pigmented extra epidermal tissues.

Table 23 *Contd...*

Sl. No	Strain identification	Generations	Characteristics of inbred strain
A	B	C	D
59.	PL/J	84	Incidence of leukemia, 80-90%, low incidence of mammary tumors.
60.	PS	38	Incidence of mammary tumors, 38% incidence of leukemia, 31% (24% lymphoid, 7% myeloid), 8 % of mammary tumors associated with leukemia, amyloidosis frequent in old mice.
61.	RF	64	Incidence of leukemia, 45-50% blood pressure & resistance of radiation in midrange, glomerulosclerosis
62.	RFM	---	Low incidence of spontaneous leukemia, differs at Es 2 locus from all other strains tested.
63.	RIII	66	High incidence of mammary tumors but varies among sublines, carries mammary tumor agent, urethane causes hepatic angiomatosis.
64.	SJL	59	Incidence of reticulum cell sarcoma 90 % both sex, incidence of hepatosplenic amyloidosis, 50% after 6 mo, low incidence of audiogenic seizures, paraproteins very elevated, high resistance to both chronic & whole body irradiation, blood pressure in midrange.
65.	SM	66	Very low incidence of any kind of tumor, incidence of amyloidoisis, 100% at 1 yr, body size small at birth & at weaning (relatively small size tends to disappear as animals mature)
66	ST/b	96	Incidence of leukemia (including some plasma cell), 1-2%, incidence of other tumors (including lung & mammary), 3%
67.	STOLI	117	Low incidence of leukemia,
68.	SWR	101	Low incidence of mammary tumors, incidence of primary lung tumor ≈ 50% female develop polydipsia at 6-10 mo, high mortality in male with vitamin-K deficiency or when exposed to oxidation products of ethylene oxide, midrange of radiation resistance, arteriosclerosis common in both sex, resting O_2 consumption highest 7 strains tested.

Table 23 *Contd...*

Sl. No	Strain identification	Generations	Characteristics of inbred strain
A	B	C	D
69.	TS	40	Useful for antibody-mediated immunosuppression study.
70.	WB	75	Homozygotes (WW) are anaemic, sterile, & lack pigmentation in coat, anemic mice die at ≈ 11 da, heterozygotes (Ww) have normal blood & fertility, but white ventral spotting.
71.	WC	70	Same as WB, except that mean age of anaemic mice at death is 14 da, some surviving to adulthood.
72.	WH	71	Same as WB, except that anaemic mice die at ≈ 5 da.
73.	WK	60	Same as WB. Except that anaemic mice die at ≈ 10 da.
74	X/Gf	52	No leukemia or solid tumors, radiation does not induce tumors, life span, 2 yr.
75.	YBR	96	Low incidence of tumors amyloidosis in at least 50% of both sex obesity in hybrids.
76.	101	61	Low incidence of mammary tumor, moderate fertility, susceptible to skin & lung-tumor induction.
77.	129/J	66	Incidence of varied types of tumor, 12% in male, 20% in virgin female, not susceptible to mammary tumor agent, highly sensitive to estrogen at all ages ; very resistant to X-radiation ; high incidence of urinary calculi: relatively low blood pressure.
78.	XVII	60	Low incidence of mammary tumor & leukemia ; incidence of pulmonary adenomas, 20% after 15 mo ; blood catalase activity low.
79.	XLII	41	Very low incidence of tumors ; hepatomas induced by radiation.

Based on "Biology Data Book" – By Philips C. Altman and Dorothy S. Ditlmer.

The Laboratory Rat▲

CLASS : Mammalia ORDER : Rodentia

FAMILY: Muridae GENUS : Rattus

SCIENTIFIC NAME: *Rattus norvegicus*

Rat is one of the most commonly and vastly used class of laboratory animals. Its popularity as laboratory animal is next only to that of mice. Just as the mice, rat's availability spreads over the whole world specially in places of human habitation. *Rattus norvegicus* adapts readily to breeding and living in the laboratory conditions. It is belived that about 3 to 5 million rats are used yearly in laboratories all over the world, which account for use of 10-15% of the total number of laboratory animals of different species. Rats are used mainly in the research of toxicity, nutrition, behaviour and cancer. A smaller number in proportion is also used in physiological investigations as well as for teaching.

Over last few decades, the laboratory rat has been developed from the wild brown rat, known as the 'Norwegian rat'. Three well-knows groups of strains as under have been developed and these groups have served as the source for the numerous substrains of rats.

Strains of Rat

1. **The Wistar Albino**

   This strain was developed originally at Wistar Institute, Phile. Delphia, U.S.A. It is a prolific strain and is now maintained in various laboratories all over the world. It is rather resistant to infections and has a low incidence of spontaneous tumors.

2. **The Sprague-Dawley Albino Rat**

   The strain was developed at Sprague-Dawley Farms, Madison, Wisconsin, U.S.A. The animals grow more rapidly and are more prolific than the Wistar. It is less resistant to infection, especially respiratory infections.

3. **The Long-Evans Rat**

   This strain is comparatively smaller in size than the Wistar and the Sprague-Dawley strains. It has a black hood over the head, black at the back of the neck and has black lines over the back. They are known also as "hooded-rats".

The Wistar albino strain has been selected as the representatives of the species for discussion.

Exterior Features of Rat

The Wister rat possesses a big sized head and long ears. The length of the tail is always shorter than the body-length. Its body is of long cylindrical stature with long thin tail and very short legs. The head has a pointed snout with two slit-like nostrils, a narrow mouth with short lower jaw and split upper lip, two small round and glistening eyes-set so that they look diagonally forward and side ways two rounded pinnac and good number of whiskers (long stiff hairs near the mouth). It has a short neck. The trunk is shortly wider than the head. The anus is at the base of the tail. In the female the urinary and genital apertures are anterior to the anus on the ventral surface of the hind and of the abdomen. The female has ten/twelve nipples, situated in two rows on either side of belly. In the male the common urogenital aperture is at the tip of the short retractile penis, behind which are two very large scrotal sacs. The body weight of an adult rat stands around 250-450 gms or more. It is about 16 cms; in length from the snout to the base of the tail which is about 12-14 cms in length.

Anatomical Peculiarities of Rat

Anatomically rats are nearly similar to mice. They can also produce gnawing due to their peculiar teeth. They do not have any vomiting centre [absence of CTZ] tonsil or gall bladder. They have extremely diffuse pancreas. The stomach shows an obvious division into two parts by a prominent white somewhat curved transverse ridge. The upper two-fifth non-secretary portion (rumen) is translucent and thinner than the lower three-fifth glandular secretory portion. The antrum is roughly semicircular area straddling the lesser curvature below the limiting ridge. It is relatively thin and translucent, and has a slightly irregular inner lining. The remainder of the lower two-third comprises the body of the stomach which straddles the entire greater curvature below the ridge except for a small area above the pylorus. This is the thick portion of the stomach with mucosa thrown into folds. This part of the stomach is analogous to the body of the stomach in man both anatomically and functionally.

Housing of Rat

The rats can be housed in the cages in the laboratory, cages being made of plastic, galvanized iron, anodised aluminium or stainless steel. The base floor of the cage can be either solid or screen bottomed. The solid bottomed cages are either placed on the shelf or suspended whereas a screen bottomed cage is always suspended. The thickness of the wire used for mesh of the screen bottom should be 0.0359 inch in diameter (20 guage) and the mesh should have 2 × 2 openings per square inch to afford maximum comfort to the animal placed on it. When screen bottomed cages are used, a shallow tray is placed underneath the cages to facilitate the collection of urine and faecal droppings. These trays can be provided with some materials which absorbs moisture to reduce bacterial growth and the resultant smell. The trays are subjected to thorough washing and disinfection everyday. Usually, some material (saw dust or rice husk is) provided as bedding inside the solid bottom cage. This provide warmth and comfort to the animal inside the cage, besides absorbing urine and moisture from the faeces. In order to ward off any chance of out break of disease, the cage and the bedding should be replaced at quick and regular intervals with provision of fresh cages with bedding.

The size of the cage will depend upon the age, size and the number of animals to be housed. The minimum recommended floor space per adult rat is 258 sq. cm and the minimum height of the cage should be 17.3 cm. A cage with a floor area of 850 sq. cm can be conveniently used to house a female with as many as 14 young with her. A breeding male and six adult females can be accommodated in a cage with a floor area of not less than 1700 sq. cm. But as the animals grow older and bigger, they will need more space for breeding.

The density of rats in a cage has a marked effect on the weight-gain of weaning rats. The young animals lose heat very rapidly if exposed in a large airy cage with too few companions for huddling. On the other hand, rats which are older than 3 weeks will not tolerate too many companions in a cage, mainly because of excessive heat production.

The Colony of Rat

For laboratory use, it is better and convenient to maintain a rat colony, although in some localities rats are adequately available for purchase from local dealers. It is advisable to begin with a good stock of rats for selection of best progency for breeders. While attaining age of six months, rats will have reached nearly their full size. Wood savings are more or less satisfactory for bedding and the cages should be cleared weekly with hot water and with 5% DDT solution once a month to prevent infections.

Requirement of External Environment of Rat

An ideal temperature for rats ranges between 20°C to 25°C but rapid and frequent fluctuations have to be avoided to prevent any injury. When the animals are caged in open wire cages, the ambient temperature should be more cautiously controlled, than if they are housed in solid walled plastic cages. The relative humidity (RH) is very critical for rats. It should be maintained anywhere between 50 - 55%. If RH falls below 45% and the temperature is also low, an out break of ring tail may crop up. Ring tail occurs in a colony where the relative humidity falls below 45% and the temperature is less than 20°C. Under this condition the new-born rats develop reddened tails that become swollen, and constricted with corrugated rings. The tail and occassionally the toes blacken and drop off. During winter season the ring tail usually occurs. A very effective ventilation system should be provided in housing since the rats are very susceptible to lung infections. In case of air-conditioned colony, twelve to fifteen change of air per hour in the animal rooms are recommended. Twelve hours of light and twelve hours of darkness should ensure optimum breeding activity. The intensity of light inside the animal rooms should be 350 - 400 lux, one metre above floor level.

Handling of Rat

Rats are more inclined to human handling, unlike the mice, rats can be tamed by soft and gentle handling. They will rarely bite unless startled or hurt. Like mice, small rats may be picked up by tail. Bigger animals can also be similarly handled for short periods, but proximal half, preferably root of the tail must be grasped. A heavy rat should not be held by its tail for longer time, since the tail skin may tear. While, however, handling the rat by tail, the animal should not be dangling in the air, as it may create panic to the animal.

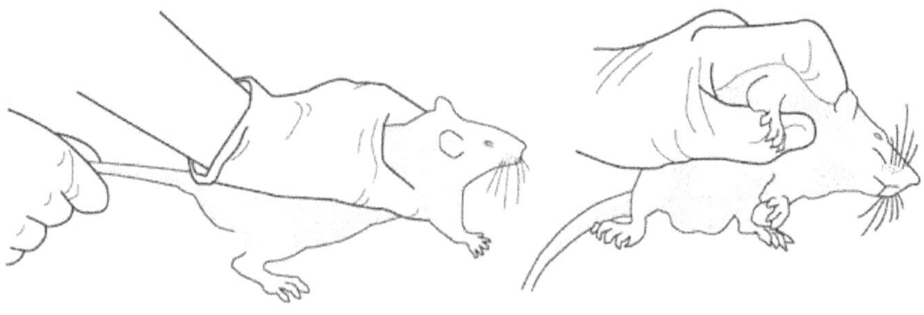

(a) (b)

Fig. 10 Holding of rat a, b.

Larger rats, especially the pregnant females should not be picked up, but only caught, by the tail. The weight should be taken by a hand, either underneath the body or by grasping the rat over the shoulder and chest. A rat will not show annoyance at if being grasped from above, but it will be nervous if driven into a corner and can attempt to bite.

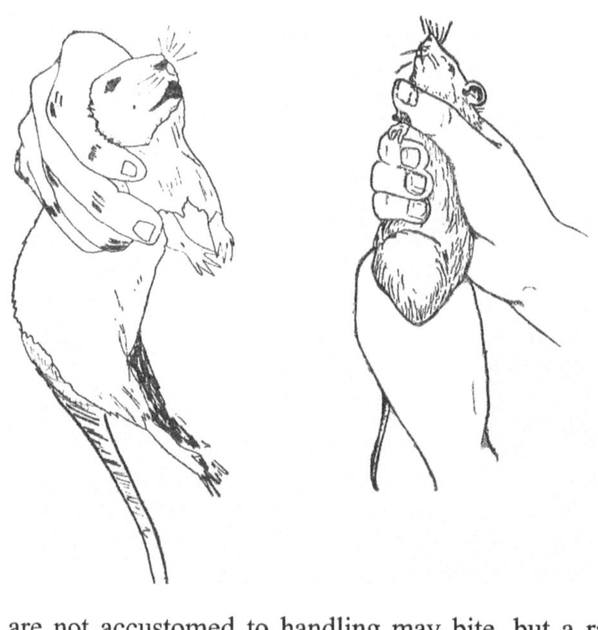

Rats, who are not accustomed to handling may bite, but a rat with his mouth shut cannot bite. Therefore, it should be caught with thumb and index finger around and below the lower jaw (not around the throat). The body or throat should not be squeezed and obviously it will struggle to escape. It is easy to pick up rats by tail, which incidentally does them no harm, because they will pull away and can be picked up while straining. They cannot be held along suspended by their tails because they will climb up and attempt to bite. Gloves can be worn but this is not convenient and also not necessary if proper handling technique is adopted.

Nutritional Requirement of Rat

Like mice, rats are omnivorous and infact, used to devour all things and are experimental feeders. Unfamiliar foods are consumed by the rats with great care and caution and return to such foods only if they have not suffered any ill effects. Their nutritional requirements would be adequately satisfied by many combinations of food stuffs. For all practical purposes, the nutritional requirements are the same as those of mice. An adult rat consumes about 12-15 gms of diet and drinks about 35 ml of water per day. Diets of highly purified ingredients, prepared in dried checker or cube form, can surely promote excellent growth and reproduction in rats. Such type of diet is formulated from food values measured in terms of proteins, fats, carbohydrates, vitamins, minerals and water. The cube method affords certain advantages. It is economical and simple to feed and handle, does not spoil, and permits ease in cage cleaning. The diet becomes actually monotonous as noticed that the rats have interest in other preferential types of food, if available for supply in cages.

Breeding of Rat

The laboratory rat is sexually mature at the age of 6 1/2 to 7 1/2 weeks. The female rats obtains her first estrus at 6 to 7 weeks of age. The testes of the male descend at about this time, but they are retractable throughout life. Rats are introduced for the first mating when they are between 90 - 120 days of age. Males and females used for mating should be approximately of the same size and age.

Age at sexual maturity (days)	Breeding seasons	Estrus		Gestation period days	Young
		Type	Cycle (days)		no/litters
45-53	all year	P	45	21	8-16

Estrus Cycle of Rat

The estrus cycle of the rat occurs usually every 4 to 5 days and each is characterized by periodic histological changes in the epithelium of the uterus and vagina.

The estrus cycle of the rat is divided into four stages according to the cell types found in the vaginal smear, These are pro-estrus, estrus, met-estrus and di-estrus. The estrus phase is characterized as the period of sexual receptivity when copulation is welcomed by the female.

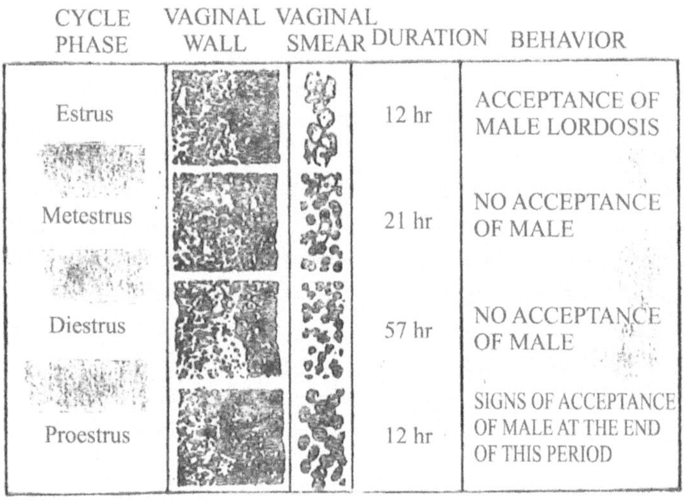

Fig. 11 Estrus Cycle of rat.

Estrus cycle does not occur when the rat is in pregnancy, pseudopregnancy or is lactating. However, soon after delivery, the female rats come into estrus, which is known as the post-partum estrus. The estrus, is followed by a period of met-estrus (which lasts for about 21 hours), di-estrus (the longest of the phases, about 57 hours) and pro-estrus (about 12 hours duration) in the order.

Changes of Vaginal Smear during an Estrus Cycle of Rat

The estrus cycle is followed by observing the changes in types of cells in the vagina, the so called *"Vaginal Smear"*. In order to elicit this smear, tufts of cotton are wrapped tightly around the ends of toothpicks, the swab moistened with saline and gently inserted and slightly rotated within the vagina. Thereafter swab pressed in a drop of saline on a glass slide and examined under low power microscope. From day to day appearance of the cells in the smear noting as well as recording is made.

During an anestrus portion of the cycle the smear consists preponderantly of leucocytes with an occasional cornified epithelial cell. The first appearance of the estrus is marked by mucification of vagina, rapidly followed by the complete or nearly complete, disappearance of leucocytes and their replacement by good numbers of round, nucleated, epithetical cells. These cells are about three times as large as the leucocytes and once seen, cannot be mistaken. At this stage, after about 12 hours, the animal will breed, but at no other time. Desquamation of the epithelial cells now occurs and white cheesy masses of disintegrating squamous cells are noticed in the smear. Leucocytes now again make their appearance and the cycle is repeated. The whole cycle in the rat last for about 5 days, being divided roughly into 3 days of anestrus and 2 days spent in the manifestation of estrus just described. The cycle appears at puberty which reaches in rats at the age of 60-90 days.

Mating Technique of Rat

Both monogamous and polygamous methods of mating (pairing with another of opposite sex) are practised in rats. With a view to having collection of a large numbers of young, two males and six females are accommodated together in one cage. The female rats remain there till pregnant. Each female rat is examined in the cage twice a week for signs of pregnancy. The presence of a droplet of blood at the vaginal opening by day 6-10th of pregnancy or a marked increase in weight approximately 25-50 gms by days 12 to 18, is indicative of pregnancy. Enlargement of abdomen and nipples is evident by 14th day of gestation. All female rats burdened with pregnancy are segregated in individual cages and remain there until the litters are born and weaned. Paper cuttings duly sterilized are spread in the cage as nesting materials.

The average periodicity of gestation is 21 days, and the maximum number of deliveries generally taking place at 22 days of gestation.

Timed Pregnancies

By dint of monitoring the estrus cycle through vaginal smears, only females in heat can be mated. Another method is to examine the females introduced for mating for the presence of copulatory plug or vaginal plug every morning. In rats, unlike in mice, the plug may fall off easily and hence may not be observed. In such cases a vaginal swab can be taken and the smear can be examined for the presence of sperms in the smear. The day on which the copulatory plug or the sperm is observed in the smear is counted as day zero of pregnancy.

The rat gives birth to 8-16 pups per delivery. The litter size may very from strain to strain depending on parity. Usually the earlier litters are large. The litter size may gradually decrease after the 6th litter. A female will bread successfully till about 14 to 16 months of age when menopause may occur. This is indicated by irregular cycles and frequent bursts of activity during the transition. During this period a maximum of litters can be produced per female breeder.

Breeding Nucleus (Foundation Stock)

It is essential to have a breeding nucleus in order to maintain a breeding colony of rats. The breeding nucleus (foundation stock) normally consists of 6 to 8 monogamous pairs of breeders. The animals for the foundation stock are selected either from existing stock or obtained from other animal colonies maintaining good quality animals of known strain. Animals for breeding nucleus are selected from litters with the following qualities, varieties or criteria

(a) Large litter size (Animals from litters having lees number of pups than average litter size are avoided).
(b) Good birth weight (above average) and more or less equal sex ratio.
(c) Least mortality between day of birth and weaning (least pre-weaning mortality).
(d) No cannibalism by mother.
(e) No abnormal pups in the litter.
(f) Good weight at weaning (above average).
(g) Consistent litter size (hence usually the animals for breeding are selected from 2nd or 3rd litter).
(h) Tameness (animals which have a tendency to bite or are aggressive are avoided from breeding stock).
(i) Early maturity (puberty and sexual maturity).

Most of the strains of rats attain sexual maturity around 90 days of age. The breeding nucleus or foundation stock animals are breed by inbreeding (brother x sister) in monogamous pairs. From each pair (usually from second or third litter) animals are chosen for next generation. The excess animals are passed on to the production colony. In the production colony animals can be breed rampantly by polygamous method. A group of 4-6 females can be mated with one male. The advanced pregnant females are separated to individual clean cages to give birth to pups. Pregnant females have to be provided with sufficient diet, water (*ad libitum*) and clean quarters. On the day of delivery the pups are seized and average weight at birth (for males and females separately) is recorded. If in any particular litter the number of pups born are less than average (say less than 8) excess pups from some other litter (born in the same day or previous day) can be nourished, so that all suckling mothers will have uniform number of pups. This will ensure more or less uniform weight at the time of weaning.

The young ones are weaned on day 21 post-partum. Each animal is weighed and the weights are recorded. They are seized and housed in groups of 3-4 in each cage, ready to be supplied for experimental work, depending upon the experimental requirement such as age and or weight-range. After weaning, each breeder is rested for 4-6 days and reintroduced for mating. In case a large number of rats are required, the females can be mated post-partum. The rats will come into estrus soon after delivery. If a male is present in the cage, then she will get mated soon after delivery (post-partum mating) thereby lactation and gestation will run concurrently.

The females have to be provided with additional dietary supplements to cope with additional stress and nutritional requirement. Generally skimmed milk powder is supplemented in the diet (2-3% extra).

By means of practising post-partum (intensive breeding), it would be possible to get a birth in course of every 21 days, But it is likely that the pups will not be as healthy as those raised from non-intensive breeding. In the process of non-intensive breeding it may be possible to get atleast 5 6 litters per breeder during its active breeding span. There may be a reduction in litter size subsequent to 4th or 5^{s} litter. Such litters are usually called off. Whenever a pregnant female is separated from the breeding group, the group size can be kept constant by introducing another female to the group. The animals weaned from the production colony are kept in the holding room on holding area, awaiting despatch for the experimental work. A schematic representation of the animals in foundation stock, production colony and the holding room is indicated hereunder:

1 **Foundation stock**	2 **Production colony**	3 **Holding colony**
6-8 monogamous pairs →	30-500 breeders depending upon the requirement of animals. → All animals produced here are supplied. The old breeder are replaced by replacement from the foundation stock.	Animals to be issued for experimental work.

Life Span of Rat

The life span of the albino rat is about 2 - 3 years. A great majority of laboratory rats develop chronic respiratory disease, which results in progressive damage to the lungs, so that by the time the animal is 1.5 to 2 years, old, a large proportion of the lungs tissue is damaged.

Anaesthesia Techniques for Rat

Usually in rat the same anaesthetic is used for induction and for maintenance and is given by injection. Experiments in which the animal recovers, however, it may be more convenient and safer to use a volatile anaesthetic. For minor surgical procedures of short duration such as cardiac puncture, carbondioxide or anaesthetic ether can be used to produce anaesthesia. Either solid carbondioxide or ether is placed in the bottom of a glass desiccator, covered with a perforated platform and the rat put in the vessel which is then closed. The animal is removed when it has lost consciousness and the operation procedure is quickly carried out. For blood sampling by means of cardiac puncture, carbondioxide anaesthesia is preferable since it causes the least change in blood chemistry.

For anaesthesia of rat, urethane is frequently used. It is convenient to give half the anaesthetic dose by the intraperitoneal (IP), route and when the animal is partly anaesthetized, to give reminder subcutaneously (SC). It may be necessary to wait 20 to 30 minutes before the rat is fully anaesthetized. This method combines the relatively rapid onset of the IP injection with more prolonged duration of SC injection. It has been found that less satisfactory results are obtained when the entire dose is given by one route.

Ether can be used for experiments of longer duration, although it does cause troublesome and copious salivary and bronchial secretions, and in addition is highly inflammable. The volatile non-inflammable anaesthetic halothane is much more suitable and with it depth of anaesthesia can be easily controlled. Recovery is very rapid without any of the side effects associated with ether anaesthesia.

Pentobarbitone sodium is quite a satisfactory alternative of urethane anaesthetic in rats for short procedures. Sodium hexobarbitone can be administered by IP, or IV route to produce short acting anaesthesia. Male rats metabolize barbiturates more rapidly than female rats and so will require even more frequent maintenance doses.

Some preparation (e.g. the pithed rat) must be ventilated artificially. In other experiments (e.g. neuromuscular blocking agents) artificial respiration might be necessary because the animal's breathing has become inadequate. The rate and volume of respiration are most important and the following are recommended : 400 ml/kg/min.

During anaesthesia it is usually necessary to warm the animal because its temperature-regulating mechanism is not functioning normally. The operating table itself may be placed on a small electric blanket. Alternatively the animal may be heated by an overhead infra-red lamp. Whatever method is used, it is important to check the rectal temperature of the animal and to see that it is maintained within normal limits i. e. 37.3° ± 0.5°C. Ideally a feedback circuit is used so that the animals temperature control the heat source and when the animal gets too cold the heat is switched on.

Collection of Blood from Rat

The composition of a blood sample will depend on the method of sampling. In long term experiments therefore, it is imperative that the same method should be adopted throughout for both control and experimental animals. Analytical methods which will enable the volume of the blood sample withdrawn, to be kept to a minimum, should be chosen.

Small blood samples can be obtained from a tail vein by snipping the tip of the tail. The animal including the tail, should be kept warm by means of a lamp and gently restrained. The tip of the tail is cleansed with alcohol and when this has dried the tip is snipped with a clean scalpel and the blood collected in a pipette or directly on to a slide or tube, after discarding the first few drops. The tail must not be massaged which can be diluted with tissue fluids.

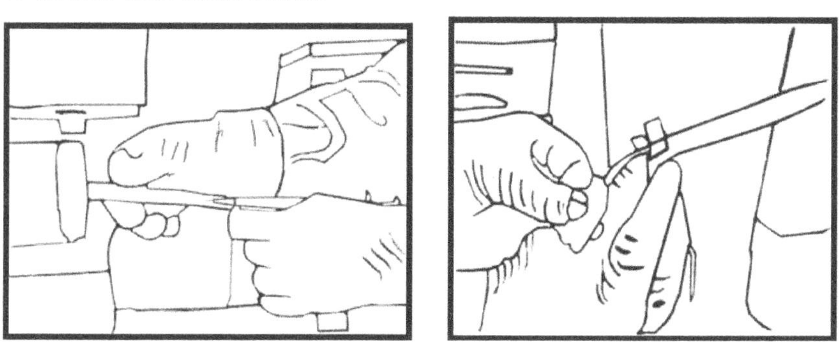

Fig. 12 Blood sample collection from rat tail vein.

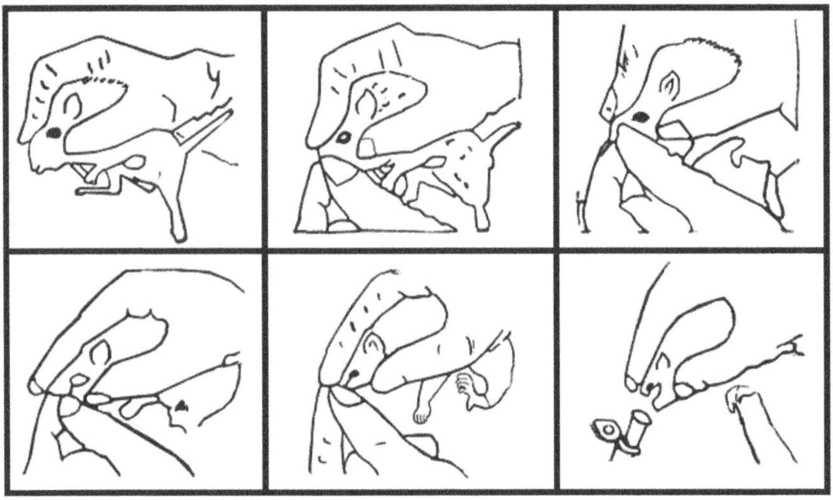

Fig. 13 Blood sample collection from rat orbital sinus.

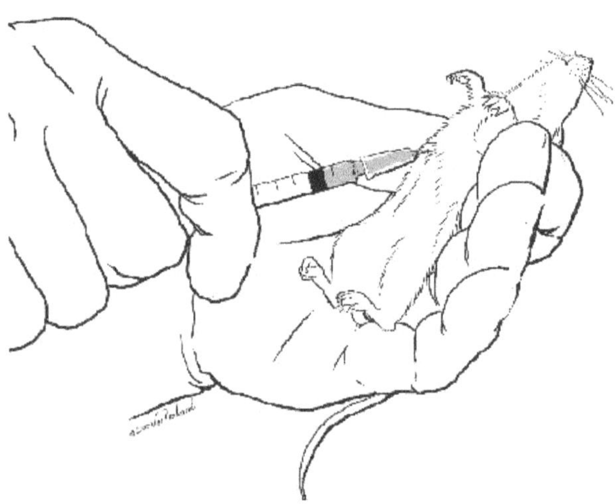

Fig. 14 Blood sample collection through cardiac puncture in rat.

Large blood samples should be collected by cardiac puncture. The anaesthetized rat is placed on its back and the heart located under the 5th or 6th rib by palpation with the index finger of the left hand, the left thumb being held on the rat's right side. A 2-5 ml capacity syringe and a 19- 25 mm 24 - 26 guage needle is suitable for the purpose. The needle is inserted at 45° to the long axis of the body into the thoracic cavity upto the point where the heart is felt throbbing against the needle. The needle is then pushed into the ventricle and blood sample is drawn. The syringe and needle can contain an anticoagulant (Heparin) if necessary. Large samples of blood can be collected from anaesthetized rats by orbital sinus with a haematocrit tube. In rat the total blood volume is about 6 - 7 % of the whole body weight. The maximum safe volume that can be collected at one bleeding is 5.5 ml/kg body-weight.

Administration of Drugs to Rats

Drugs can be administered to rat by oral (PO), subcutaneous (SC). intramuscular (IM), intraperitoneal (IP) and intravenous (IV) routes. Volumes for injections should be kept between 0.2-0 3 ml/100 gms of body weight. The dorsal tarsal vein is useful for injection as also the saphenous vein where it crosses the leg above the hock. IV injections are best given in the tail vein using a 12.7 mm × 24 guage needle. Tail veins are not readily seen as in mouse. For visibility of the veins, the tail should be dipped in saturated sodium sulphide solution for 2 minutes.

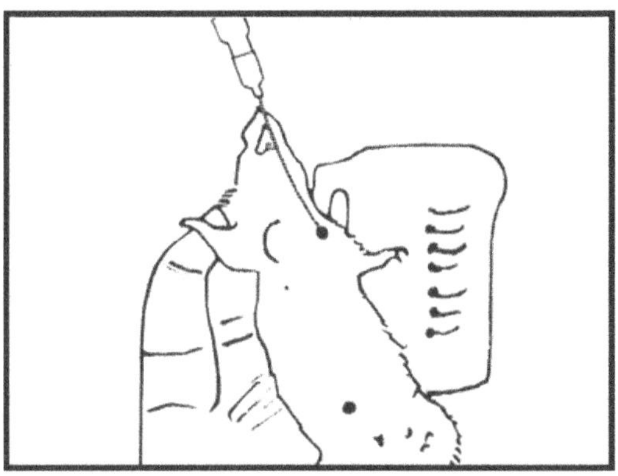

Fig. 15 (A) Oral gavage of rat.

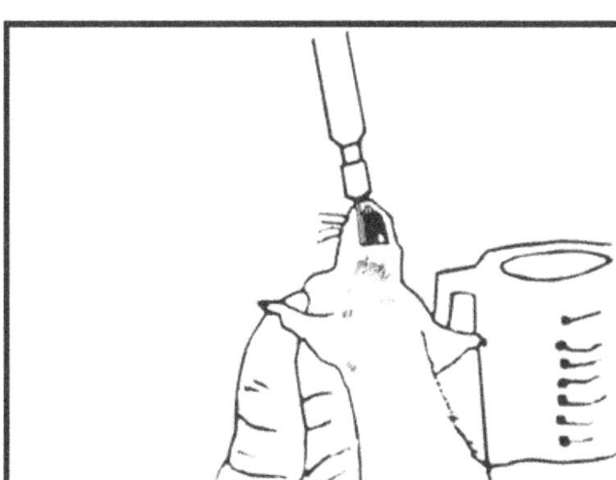

Fig. 15 (B) Oral gavage of rat.

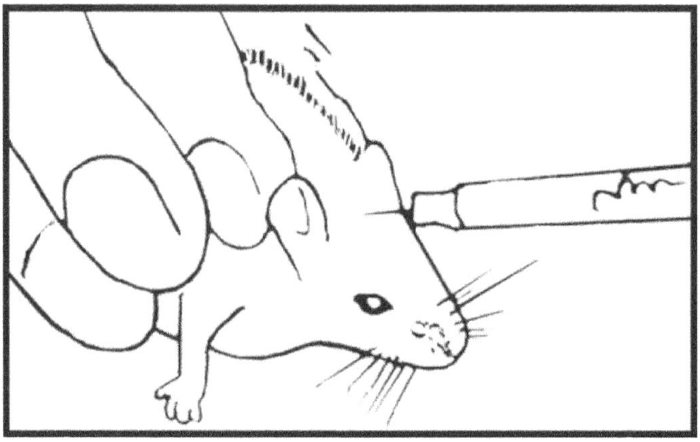

Fig. 16 Subcutaneous injection(Rat)

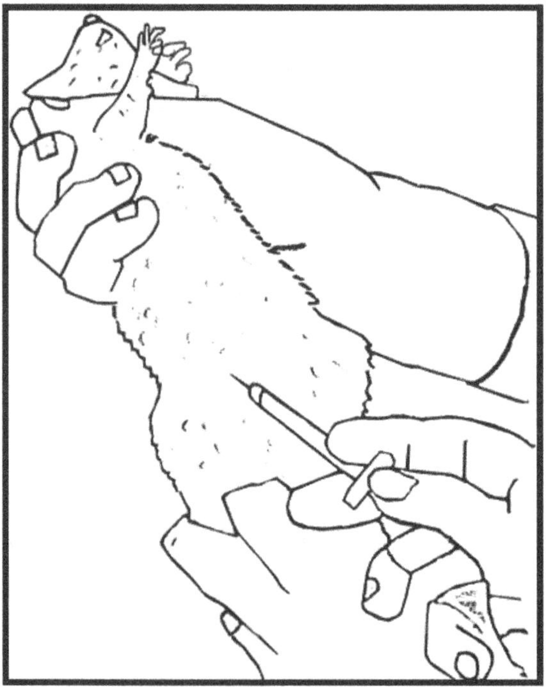

Fig. 17 Intraperitoneal injection(Rat).

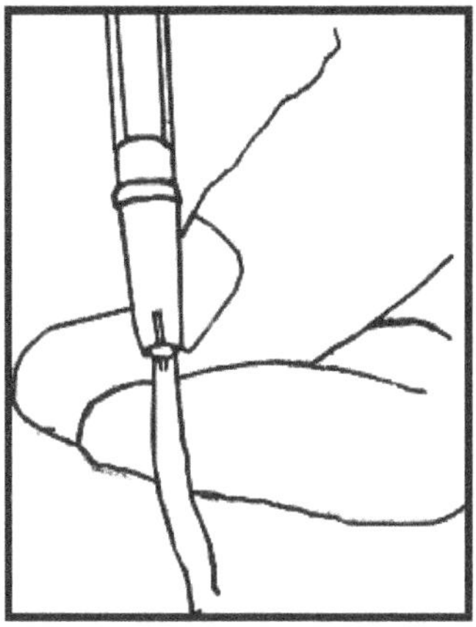

Fig. 18 Intravenous injection to a rat.

PO injection is made with a syringe fitted with a long hypodermic needle with a bulb soldered on to the top end. This needle is inserted into the mouth and gently slid over the tongue and pushed downwards. It should slide easily into stomach passing through oesophagus. If there is any resistance the needle should be withdrawn and another attempt is made to find the oesophageal opening. It is helpful to lift the rat's head slightly to align the oesophageal and stomach orifices.

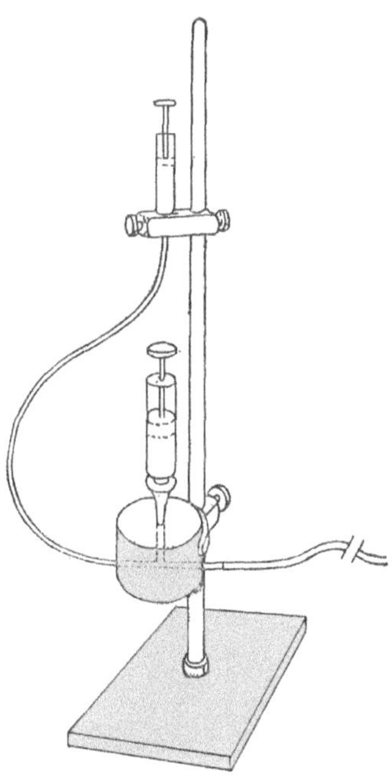

(a)

Fig. 19 Apparatus for repeated I.V. injections to rat, a, b.

Common Diseases of Rat

In general rat is quite resistant to infections. However, some diseases of bacterial, viral and parasitic origin are known to appear, even in well maintained rat colonies. These infections can be eliminated by early detection. In practice, a disease contracted animal should be destroyed. Rat is very much susceptible to respiratory infections.

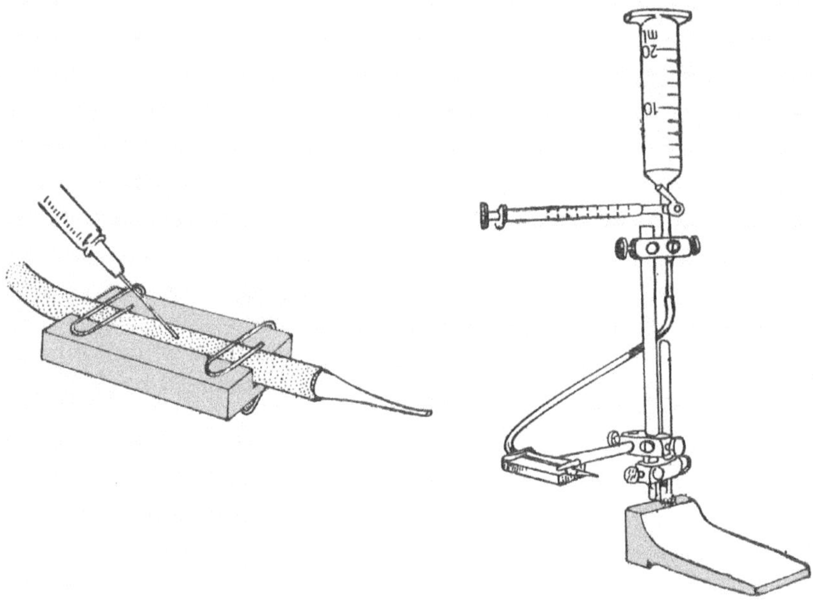

(b)

An affected rat will start losing weight and produce characteristic wheezing or chattering noise. The hair coat will be staring and there will be increased respiration.

Euthanasia of Rat

Ether or carbondioxide in a jar can be used to kill a rat without pain or discomfort. Sodium pentobarbitone injected intraperitoneally at three times the anaesthetic dose can also be applied.

DATA RELATED TO RATS

(Tables)

Table 1 Some Important Biological and Physiological Data of Rat

Mature weights		Birth Weight (gms.)	Weaning weight (gms.)	Weaning age (days)	Life span (yrs.)	Age suitable for experimentation (mos.)	Sexual maturity (days)	Time of ovulation from on set of estrus hrs.)	First mating age days	Breading habit (male to number of female)	Duration of sexual life (mos.)	Rest period of female between matings (days)
Male (gms.)	Fe-male (gms.)											
250-450	180-350	5-6	35-45	21-23	2-3	1,5	45-53	8-11	90-120	5	14-16	15
Eyes open (days)	**Ears open (days)**	**Incision erupt (days)**	**Young finds way to mother (days)**	**Hair obscures nipple in female (days)**	**Hair obscures genitalia (days)**	**First molar erupts (days)**	**Second molar erupts (days)**	**Third molar erupts (days)**	**Testes descend (days)**	**Vagina opens (days)**	**Begins eating solid food (days)**	**Menopause occurs (days)**
12-13	2.5-3.5	8-10	9-11	16	16	19	21	35	4.-45	45-50	14-15	450-470

Table 2 Milk: Composition of Rat

Water (%)	Fat (%)	Protein (%)	Sugar (%)
70-74	10-15	7-12	3.0-3.5

Based on LIAS Centre News.

Table 3 Blood Pressure of Rats

Systolic (mm. Hg)	Diastolic (mm. Hg)
116	90

Table 4 Heart Rate of Rat

Specification	
Body weight (gms.)	**Beats/min**
Normal	362
Bambro	(92-256)
New born	161 (121-201)
Young	(500-525)
252 g ; anesthetized	352 (260-450)
272 g ; 36.9°C ; anesthetized	(330-480)

Table 5 Oxygen Consumption of Rat

Body weight (gm.)	Temperature °C		O_2 Consumption ml./gm/hr.	Deviation (%)
	Body	Ambient		
545	37.5	28	0.84	+ 15

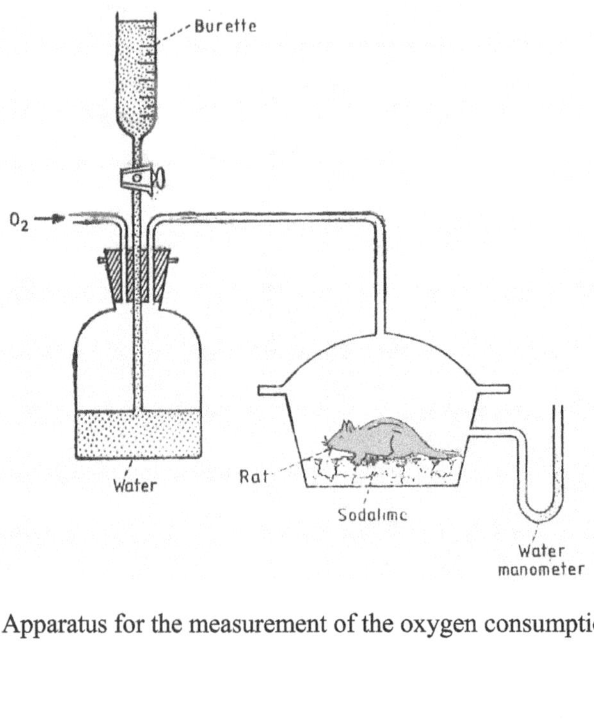

Fig. 20 Apparatus for the measurement of the oxygen consumption of rat

Table 6 Respiratory Frequency, Tidal Volume and Minute Volume of Rat

Body weight (kg)	Condition of animal	Respiratory Frequency breaths/min.	Tidal volume (ml.)	Minute volume ltrs/min.
0.113 (0.06-0.152)	Normal	85.5 (66-114)	0.86 (0.60-1.25)	0.73 (0.05-0.101)

Table 7 Dimension of Lung Respiratory Zones of Rat

Specification *	(Morphological Parameters) Values
A	B
Wt, (kg)	0.14 ± 0.007
VL, (ml)	6.3 ± 0.2
Sa, (m^2)	0.39 ± 0.02
Sc, (m^2)	0.41 ± 0.02
Vc, (ml)	0.48 ± 0.02
τ, (μm)	1.42 ± 0.07
τht, (μm)	0.38 ± 0.02
τhp, (μm)	0.18 + 0.005
τtmin	0.15
DLmax	0.83 ± 0.03
Sc : Sa ;	1.05
V_c/Sa, (ml/m^2)	1.23

* Previously expressed.

Table 8 Erythrocyte and Hemoglobin Values of Rat

Erythro-cyte count millions/μl. blood	Erythro-cyte Packed volume ml/100 ml. blood	Erythro-cyte Volume (μ^3)	Haemoglobin concentration		Erythro-cyte Haemo-globin content (pg)	Erythro-cyte Dimen-sions(μ)
			gms/ 100ml blood	gms/ 100ml RBC		
8.9 (7.2-9.6)	46 (39-53)	61 (57-65)	14.8 (12.0 -17.5)	32 (30-35)	17 (15-19)	7.5 (6.0-7.5)

Table 9 Leukocyte Counts of Rat

Leukocytes Total	Neutrophil	Eosino-phils	Basophils	Lypho-cytes	Monocytes
Thousands /µl. of blood	Thousands /µl. of blood	Thousands /µl. of blood	Thousands /µl of blood	Thousands /µl of blood	Thousands /µl. of blood
14.0 (5.0-25.0)	3.1(1.1-6.0) 22 (9-34)%	0.3 (0-0.7) 2.2 (0-6)%	0.1 (0-0.2) 0.5 (0-1.5)%	10.2 (7.0-16.0) 73 (65-84)%	0.3 (0-0.65) 2.3 (0-5)%

Note: % of total leukocytes

Table 10 Blood Platelet Counts of Rat

Platelets thousands/µl. of blood	Method used for estimation
1240 (1100-1380)	Direct method, phase microscopy

Table 11 Blood Carbohydrate of Rat

Age and Conditions	Blood Component	Carbohydrate Estimated	Concentration mg/100 ml	Method of Carbohydrate Estimation
Adult	Erythrocyte	Glucuronic acid	0 4 (0-1.0)	Naphthoresorcinol
Adult	Plasma	Glucuronic acid	0.9 (0.5-1.1)	Naphthoresorcinol
Adult, fasted 18 hrs.		Pentoses. (total)	5.27 (5.05-5.44)	Meybaum (Modification)
Adult, (19 da pregnant) fed ad lib		Glucose	80.9 ± 2.8	Glucose oxidase
Fasted 48 hr.			51.3 ± 3.2	Glucose oxidase
Adult, kept at 22°C (15 : 12 light dark regimen)	Whole Blood	Glucose	94.2 ± 4.6 (55-140)	Ferriferro cyanide
Adult, kept at 4°C (12:12 light : dark regimen)			92.0 ± 3.5 (64-127)	Ferriferrocyanide.

Table 12 Blood Lipids of Rat

Age	Blood Component	Lipids	Concentration mg/ 100 ml.
Adult	Serum	Cholesterol, total Triglyceride Phospholipid	(120-135) (40-50) (70-125)

Table 13 Acid-Base Balance of Blood and Plasma of Rat

Part I Blood

Age	Temp. °C	Erythrocyte Packed volume ml/100 ml blood	Hb concentration Mmole/ltr.	Po_2 mm Hg	Pco_2 mm Hg
Adult	38.6	46	9.0	N. A.	(35-49)

Part II. Plasma*

Age	Temp °C	pH	Total CO_2 concentration Mmole/ltr.	HCo_3^- Concentration Mmole/ltr.	Na^+ Concentration Mmole/ltr.	Cl^- Concen-tration Mmole/ltr.
Adult	38.2	(7.26-7.44)	(20.0-28.0)	22.8	(135-155)	(99-112)

* Corrected for trapped plasma by a factor of 0.94.

Table 14 Blood Volumes of Rat

Erythrocyte Volume (ml./kg.)		Plasma Volume (ml./kg.)	Venus-Hematocrit	Whole Blood Volume (mg/kg.)	
Method	Value		% cells	Method	Value
32p	23.7 (18.4-26.0)	40.4 (36.3-45.3)	*50.3 (42.3-61.5)	*VP + VRBC	64.1 (57.5-69.9)

* Blood from carotid artery or tall vein.

Table 15 Blood Electrolytes of Rat

Blood Component	Constituent	Concentration
Plasma	Calcium	40.0 ± 0.63 meq/ltr.
	Chloride	96.2 ± 6.39 meq/ltr.
	Phosphorus	7.29 ± 0.97 mg/100 ml.
	Potassium	2.70 ± 0.16 meq/ltr.
	Sodium	118.29 ± 11.09 meq/ltr.

Table 16 Blood Non-Protein Nitrogenous substance of Rat

Age	Blood Component	Constituent	Concentration (mg/100ml. blood)
A	B	C	D
Adult	Plasma Whole blood	Urea Glutathione (reduced)	34 40 (30-45)
	Whole blood	Amino acids	
		Alanine	12.3 (8.9-15.7)
		Tryptophan	1.57 (1.5-2.0)
	Plasma	Amino acids	
		Arginine	3.2 (2 35-4 07)
		Glycine	2.27 (1.85-2.69)
		Histidine	0.92 (0.85-1.09)
		Isoleucine	1.32 (0.96-1.68)
		Leucine	2.66 (2.20-3 12)
		Lysine	5.8 (4.4-7.2)

Table 17 Monoamines of Brain Tissue of Rat

GABA (μg/gm of brain tissue)	NA (μg/gm of brain tissue)	A (μg/gm of brain tissue)	DA (μg/gm of brain tissue)	5HT (μg/gm of brain tissue)
0.33 ± 0.04	0.14 ± 0.01	0.36 ± 0.04	0.11 ± 0.02	0.52 ± 0.02

Table 18 Liver Function Tests of Rat

Cholesterol (mg/100ml. blood)	Bilirubin Conjugated (mg/100ml. blood)	Bilirubin Total (mg/100ml. blood)	SGO-T (Unit/ ml. Serum)	SGP-T (Units/ml. Serum)	ALK-phosphatase (Units/ml. Serum)	Acid Phosphatase (Units/ ml, Serum)
127.5 ± 2.00	0.48 ± 0.15	0.48 ± 0.10	89.4 ± 3.4	33.2 ± 1.8	455 ± 9.80	0.62 ± 0.03

Table 19 Renal Function Tests of Rat

Specification	Age, Condition	Value
A	B	C
Creatinine clearance, ml/min	Adult	10.1 (6.3-15.2)
ml/min./kg.	Adult	3.2 (2.2-4.2)
Cr Ethylenediaminete-traacetic acid/ml./min.	Mannitol diuresis	12.4 (8.4-20.7)
	Saline diuresis	13.9 (9.0-24.5)

Table 19 *Contd...*

Specification	Age, Condition	Value
A	B	C
Aminohippurate clearance, ml./min	Adult	60.1 (21.5-199.0)
Diodone clearance, ml./min	N.S.	36.2 (30.9-45.7)
Lodohippurate clearance, sodium/ml./min.	Mannitol diuresis	45.8 (28.0-76.2)
	Saline diuresis	55.9 (37.9-90.7)
Urea clearance, ml./min./m^2	N.S.	25.5
	Young adult	14.3 (3-28)
Tabular maxima, Diodone ml./min./m.^{2}	N.S.	33.4(29.1-37.7)
Glucose ml./min./m^2	N.S.	78.7 (51.9-105.5)
Inulin clearance, ml./min.	3 wks.	0.7 (10.39-1.03)
	4-5 wks	1.46 (0.96-1.96)
	7 wks	2.28 (1.04-3.52)
	10 wks.	2.93 (1.39-4.47)
	13 wks.	3.29 (2.19-4.39)
	Adult	0.36 (2.19-4.39)
Inulin clearance, ml./min/kg	Adult (1.0-1.5 ml-/hr-urine flow)	3.2 (1.1-4.7)
ml./hr/100 gms.	2 days	7.1(2.5-11.7)
Body wt.	4 days	13.8 (8.2-19.4)
	12-13 days	21.7 (17.7- 25.7)
	16-19 days	27.9 (16.5-39.3)
µl/min/gm	1-3 days	44.7 (0.7- – 88.7)
Kidney wt.	8-10 days	159 (63-25.5)
	16-18 days	327 (180-474)
Creatinine clearance, ml/min./kg	Adult (1.0-1.5 ml/hr urine flow)	3.1 (2.0-4.9)
P – Aminohippurate clearance	N.S.	6.2 (5.34-6. 96)
ml/min	Adult	2.31 (1.95-2.63)
ml/min/kg.	Adult	15.7 (10.0-24.8)
µl/min/gm	1-3 days	355 (99-612)
Kidney wt.	8-10 days	618 (246-990)
	16-18 days	936 (742-1130)
P – Aminohippurate extraction ratio, %	1-3 days	21.3 (10.7-31.9)
	8-10 days	40.4 (32.4-48.4)
	16-18 days	73.9 (63.7-84.1)

Table 19 *Contd...*

Specification	Age, Condition	Value
A	B	C
P – Aminohippurate clearance, corrected for extraction ratio, μl/min/g kidney wt.	1-3 days	1670 (1080-2260)
	8-10 days	1521(698-2344)
	16-18 days	1267 (995-1539)
Diodone clearance ml/min/kg	Adult	22.2 (16.6-27.8)
Urea clearance, ml./min./m^2	Adult	10.9(4.7-17.1)
Mannitol Learance ml/min./kg.	Adult	5.5 (3.8-7.2)
Filtration fraction,	N. S.	0.17 (0.10-0.24)
C_1/C_{PAH}	Adult	0.16(0.11-0.21)
Filtration fraction corrected for p – aminohippurate extraction ration, C/c_1 pAH/E_{PAH}	1-3 days	0.03 (0-0.07)
	8-10 days	0.10 (0.04-0.16)
	16-18 days	0.26 (0.14-38)
Tubular maxima p-Aminohippurate mg/min.	Adult	0.10 (0.08-0.12)
Diodone, mg./min./kg.	N.S.	1.32 (0.96-1.68) 1.86 (1.6-2.1)
Glucose, mg/min.	8 wks.	5.17 (3.11-7.23)
	13 wks,	15.3 (10.9-19.7)
Ammonia excretion after acid load, μ mole/hr 100 gms. Body wt.	9 days	12.2 (11.4-13.0)
	14 days	11.1 (6.54-15.66)
	16 days.	27.3 (3.3-51.3)
	21 days.	39.0 (27.6-50.4)
	Adult	37.2 (23.6-50.8)
Titratable acid excretion after acid load μeq/hr./100 gms. body wt.	9 days	4.12 (1.32-6.92)
	14 days	8.62 (4.26-12.98)
	16 days	16.4 (6.0-26.8)
	21 days	15.1 (0-31.9)
	Adult	4.5 (8.9-20.1)
Maximum depression of urine pH after acid load, pH	9 days	5.8 (5.0-6.6)
	14 days	6.0 (5.6-6.4)
	16 days	6.0 (5.6-6.4)
	21 days	5.9
	Adult	6.2 (5.8-6.6)
Maximum urine Osmolality after 8-hr fast, mole/ltr.	10 days	938 (762-114)
	20 days	1449 (1023-1875)

Table 20 Excretion Products in Urine of Rats

Constituents	Value (mg / kg bodywt/day)
A	**B**
Guanine	Unspecified
1-Methylguanine	Unspecified
7-Methylguanine	Unspecified
N^2-Dimethylguanine	Unspecified
Cyclic guanosine monophosphate (Guanosine-3' 5'-monophosphate)	0.04
Xanthine	Unspecified
Hypoxanthine	Unspecified
1-Methylhypoxanthine	Unspecified
Uric acid	(8-12)
Deoxycytidine	(0.091-1.818)
2-Methyl-4-amino-5-hydroxymethyl pyrimidine	Unspecified
Indole derivatives Indican, methabolic (Indoxylsulphuric acid)	Unspecified
Indoleacetic acid	Unspecified
Indoleaceturic acid	Unspecified
Indole-3-carboxylic acid	Unspecified
5-Oxyindoleacetic acid	Unspecified
Skatoxylsulphuric acid	Unspecified
Miscellaneous Allantoin	(100-600)
4-Amino-5-imidazolecarboxamide	72*
Ammonia	80
Creatine	(0-13)
Creatinine	(24-40)
Hippuric acid	16.06 (6.67-23.33)
Stamine	(20-200)*
Homovanillic acid	31*
Urea	(100-1600)
Steroid hormones:	
Androgens	18*
Enzymes	
Lactate dehydrogenase	Unspecified
Isocitrate dehydrogenase (Isocitric acid dehydrogenase)	Unspecified
Glutamate dehydrogenase	Unspecified
Cholinesterase	Unspecified

Table 20 *Contd...*

Constituents	Value (mg / kg bodywt/day)
A	B
Alkaline phosphatase	Unspecified
Acid phosphatase	Unspecified
β - Glucosidase	Unspecified
β – Galactosidase	Unspecified
Chitobiase (N – Acetyl β – Glucosaminidase)	Unspecified
β – Glucuronidase	Unspecified
Oxytocic esterase	Unspecified
Organic acid :	
Acetic acid	30
cis- Aconite acid	5
Citric & isocitric acids	25
Fumaric acid	6
α – Ketoglutaric acid	7
Lactic acid	3
Phenol (Carbolic acid)	(6-60)
Succinic acid	4
Electrolytes :	
Beryllium	Unspecified
Calcium	(3-9)
Chlorine	(50-75)
Phosphorus	30
Potassium	(50-60)
Sodium	110
Sulphur, neutral	(7-20)
Bicarbonate	6
Vitamins :	
Thiamine	(3-13)*
Riboftavin	(40-80)*
Niacin	(90-120)*
Trigonelline	(300-700)*
Niacinamide	(200-700)*
N' – Methylnicotinamide	(900-5000)*
6-Hydroxynicotinic acid	Unspecified
6-Hydroxynicotinamide	Unspecified
Pantothenic acid	(300-600)*
Vitamin B_{12} (Cobalmin)	0.203*
Ascorbic acid	(1000-6000)

Table 20 *Contd...*

Constituents	Value (mg / kg bodywt/day)
A	**B**
Carbohydrate derivatives :	
Hexosamine Mucopolysaccharides	(2.4-7.2)
Total	135 (93-177)
Nonsulphated	80 (27-132)
Sulphated	55 (24-87)
Sialic acid	(3.6-9.6)
Nitrogenous substances :	
Nitrogen, total	(200-1000)
Ammonia	(10-30)
Amino acids :	
Alanine	Unspecified
Arginine, Total	2.7
Free	1.3
Aspartic acid. Free	290*
Citruline	(0.54-2.50)
Cystine, total	500*
Glutamic acid, total	7.1
Glycine, total	6.9
Histidine, total	1-5
Free	430*
Hydroxyproline	61
Isoleucine, total	2.2
Free	430
Leucine free	2.4
Lysine, total	4.6
Free	1.0
Methionine, free	400*
Methylhistidine	Unspecified
Phenylalanine, free	800
Taurine	(5-31)
Theonine, total	2.9
Free	630*
Tryptophan, free	470*
Tyrosine, free	470*
Valine, free	930*
Purines, pyrimidines, & derivatives :	
Adenosine - 3', 5'- monophophate (Cyclic adenosine monophosphate)	(20-70)*

** **Urine Specification:** Clear yellow, p H 7.3 – 6.5, Urine out put 11 – 15 ml/day, specific gravity 1.040 – 1.076.

* μg/kg body wt/day.

* expressed as μg uronic acid/kg body wt/day.

Table 21 Chemical Composition of Nervous Tissue of Rat

Tissue specification A	**Age** **B**	**Chemical Constituent** **C**	**Concentration** **D**
Whole brain	Adult	H_2O	78% by wt.
		Cl	33 μ moles/gm
		P	98 μ moles/gm
		K	89 μ moles/gm
		Na	50 μ moles/gm
		Phosphatidal choline	0.2 mg/gm
		Phosphatidyl choline	19 mg/gm
		Phosphatidal ethanolamine	10 mg/gm
		Phosphatidyl ethanolamine	8.3 mg/gm
		Phosphatidal serine	6.5 mg/gm
		Sphingomyelin	2.9 mg/gm
		Phosphatidyl inositols	3 mg/gm
		Cerebroside	18 mg/gm
		Sulfatide	3.8 mg/gm
		Cholesterol	16 mg/gm
Myelin		H_2O	400 mg/gm
		Phosphatidal choline	34 mg/gm
		Phosphatidyl choline	15 mg/gm
		Phosphatidal ethanolamine	17 mg/gm
		Phosphatidyl ethanolamine	66 mg/gm
		Phosphatidal & Phosphatidyl serine	29 mg/gm
		Sphingomyelin	16 mg/gm
		Phosphatidyl inositols	8.4 mg/gm
		Cerebroside	67 mg/gm
		Salfatide	16 mg/gm
		Sterol	78 mg/gm
		Protein	150-290 mg/gm
Cortex		H_2O	800 mg/gm
		Phospholipid	45 mg/gm
		Glycolipid	12 mg/gm
		Sterol	9.4 mg/gm
		Protein	130 mg/gm*
White matter		H_2O	79% by wt.
Gray matter		H_2O	81% by wt.
		Cl	30 μ moles/gm
		K	98 μ moles/gm

* Estimated by difference of dry weight minus total lipids.

Table 21 *Contd...*

Tissue specification A	Age B	Chemical Constituent C	Concentration D
		Na	42 μ mole/gm
Cerebrum		Alanine	0.67 μ mole/gm
		Arginine	0.11 μ mole/gm
		Aspartic acid	2.4 μ moles/gm
		L-Cystathionine	0.015 μ mole/gm
		Cysteine	0.012 μ mole/gm
		Glutamic acid	12 μ mole/gm
		Glycine	0.63 μ mole/gm
		Histidine	0.066 μ mole/gm
		Isoleucine	0.025 μ mole/gm
		Leucine	0.064 μ mole/gm
		Lysine	0.12 μ mole/gm
		Methionine	0.037 μ mole/gm
		Ornithine	0.02 μ mole/gm
Cerebrum		Phenylalanine	0.05 μ mole/gm
		Serine & paragine	1.2 μ mole/gm
		Taurine	7.6 μ mole/gm
		Threonine & glutamine	2.4 μ mole/gm
		Tyrosine	0.078 μ mole/gm
		Valine	0.083 μ mole/gm
		γ – Aminobutyric acid	2.3 μ mole/gm
		Ammonia	0.99 μ mole/gm
		Ehanolamine	0.11 μ mole/gm
		Glutathione	1.1 μ mole/gm
		Glycerophosphoethan olamine	0.40 μ mole/gm
		Homocarnosine	0.1 μ mole/gm
		Phosphoethanolamine	2.2 μ mole/gm
Pons		Alanine	0.56 μ mole/gm
		Arginine	0.2 μ mole/gm
		Aspartic acid	2.7 μ mole/gm
		Citrulline	0.14 μ mole/gm
		L – Cystathionine	0.053 μ mole/gm

Table 21 *Contd...*

Tissue specification A	Age B	Chemical Constituent C	Concentration D
		Cysteine	0.06 μ mole/gm
		Glutamic acid	6.9 μ mole/gm
		Glutamine	0.77 μ mole/gm
		Glycine	3.5 μ mole/gm
		Histidine	0.044 μ mole/gm
		Isoleucine	0.034 μ mole/gm
		Leucine	0.064 μ mole/gm
		Lysine	0.44 μ mole/gm
		Methionine	0.043 μ mole/gm
		Ornithine	0.051 μ mole/gm
		Phenylalanine	0.05 μ mole/gm
		Serine & asparagine	0.63 μ mole/gm
Pons		Taurine	2.0 μ mole/gm
		Threonine & glutamine	1.6 μ mole/gm
		Tyrosine	0.059 μ mole/gm
		Valine	0.52 μ mole/gm
		γ – Aminobutyric acid	1.8 μ mole/gm
		Ammonia	0.89 μ mole/gm
		Ethanolamine	0.18 μ mole/gm
		Glutathione	0.62 μ mole/gm
		Glycerophosphoethan olamine	0.60 μ mole/gm
		Homocarnosine	0.059 μ mole/gm
		Phosphoethanolamine	0.51 μ mole/gm
Astrocytoma		Alanine	2.7 μ mole/gm
		- Alanine	0.029 μ mole/gm
		Arginine	0.18 μ mole/gm
		Asparagine	0.44 μ mole/gm
		Aspartic acid	0.60 μ mole/gm
		Citrulline	0.02 μ mole/gm
		L – Cystathionine	0.01 μ mole/gm
		Cysteine	0.058 μ mole/gm
		Glutamic acid	3.00 μ mole/gm

Table 21 *Contd...*

Tissue specification A	Age B	Chemical Constituent C	Concentration D
		Glutamine	0.72 μ mole/gm
		Glycine	5.5 μ mole/gm
		Histidine	0.22 μ mole/gm
		Hydroxyproline	0.01 μ mole/gm
		Isoleucine	0.18 μ : mole/gm
		Leucine	0.29 μ mole/gm
		Lysine	0.61 μ mole/gm
		Methionine	0.02 μ mole/gm
		Ornithine	0.01 μ mole/gm
		Phenylalanlne	0.17 μ mole/gm
Astrocytoma		Proline	0.85 μ mole/gm
		Serine	2.3 μ mole/gm
		Taurine	1.5 μ mole/gm
		Threonine	0.0 μ mole/gm
		Tyrosine	0.19 μ mole/gm
		Valine	0.12 μ mole/gm
		γ – Aminobutyric acid	0.14 μ mole/gm
		Ammonia	2.8 μ mole/gm
		Ethanolamine	0.12 μ mole/gm
		Glutathione	1.2 μ mole/gm
		Glycerophosphoethan olamine	0.55 μ mole/gm
		Phosphoethanolamine	3.1 μ mole/gm
		Urea	3.6 μ mole/gm
Spinal cord		Phosphatidal & phosphatidyl choline	21 mg/gm
		Phosphatidal & phosphatidyl ethanolamine	39 mg/gm
		Sphingomyelin	18 mg/gm
		Cerebroside	42 mg/gm
		Cholesterol	36 mg/gm
Microsomes		Phosphatidal & phosphatidyl choline	120 mg/gm*
		Phosphatidal & phosphatidyl ethanolamine	116 mg/gm*
		Phosphatidal & phosphatidyl serine	39 mg/gm*

Table 21 *Contd...*

Tissue specification A	Age B	Chemical Constituent C	Concentration D
		Sphingomyelin	27 mg/gm*
		Phosphatidyl inositols	14 mg/gm*
		Cerebroside	39 mg/gm*
		Sulfatide	5 mg/gm*
		Cholesterol	134 mg/gm*
Mitochondria		Phosphatidal & phosphatidyl choline	113 mg/gm*
		Phosphatidal & phosphatidyl ethanolamine	55 mg/gm*
		Phosphatidal & phosphatidyl serine	16 mg/gm*
		Sphingomyelin	25 mg/gm*
		Phophatidyl Inositols	9 mg'gm*
		Cerebroside & sulfatide	22 mg/gm*
		Cholesterol	51 mg/gm*
Nerve ending particles *		Phosphatidal & phosphatidyl choline	15 mg/gm*
		Phosphatidal & phosphatidyl ethanolamine	8.3 mg/gm*
		Phosphatidal & phosphatidyl serine	2.3 mg/gm*
		Sphingomyelin	3.3 mg/gm*
		Phosphatidyl inositols	1.1 mg/gm*
		Cerebroside & sulfatide	3.9 mg/gm*
		Cholesterol	97 mg/gm*

* Subcellular Organelle

* Dry weight.

Table 22 Tolerance to Temperature Extremes of Rat

Age Body Weight	Temperature Measured	Tolerance Limit				
		Extreme	Temp. °F	Duration	Survival	Remarks
A	B	C	D	E	F	G
Adult	Air	Upper	40	213 ± 36 mins	All survived	Heated room
			(42-43) 15	144 ± 12 mins.	All survived	
			(49-51)	31 ± 1	All survived	
60 days old	Air	Lower	2	8 days	All survived	
60 days old	Air	Lower	2	90 days	few dead	
120 days old	Air	Lower	2	25 days	All survived	
120 days old	Air	Lower	2	60 days	All survived	
227 gms	Water	Lower	20	2 hrs.	All survived	Subjects conscious at end of test.
			10	20 mins	All survived	Serious impairment, approaching unconciousness
			0	10 mins	All survived	Serious impairment, approaching unconsciousness.
235 gms	Air	Lower	– 35	0.75-2 hrs.	All dead	Cold chamber wind, 2ml/hr.
250 gms	Air	Lower	– 40	20 mins.	All dead	Summer; estimated from O_2 consumption.
280 gms	Air	Lower	– 60	20 mins.	All dead	Winter ; estimated from O_2 consumption.
280/350 gms	Air	Lower	– 18	200 mins.	All dead	Acclimated to 30°C
			– 29	200 mins.	All dead	Acclimated to 20°C
			– 35	200 mins.	All dead	Acclimated to 10°C

Table 23 Typical Electroencephalograms of Rat

Age	Experimental conditions	Frequency (H_z)	Amplitude (μV)	Remarks
Adult	Alert	10-30	–	"Activated" sleep
	Relaxed-asleep	2-10	–	
	Alert	8-16	50-100	"Activated" sleep; cortical theta
	Relaxed-asleep	2-8	100-200	
	Alart	30-40	30	"Activated" sleep; cortical theta
	Relaxed-asleep	2-6	50-75	Subtle difference in frequency between alert condition and "activated" sleep.

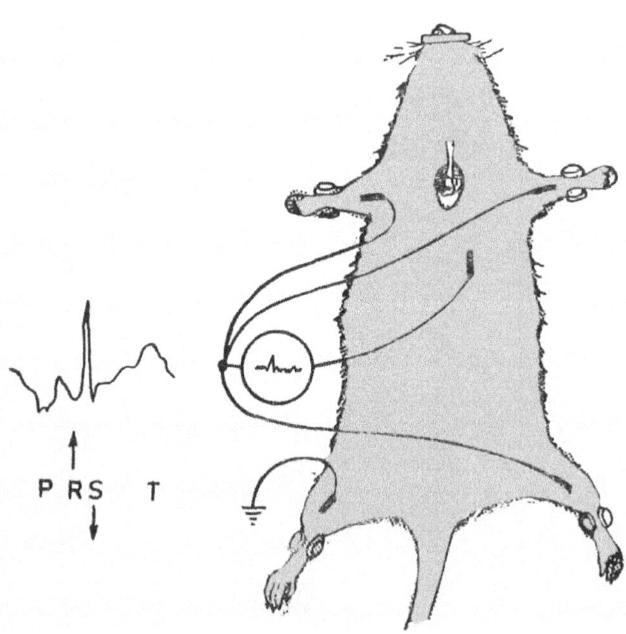

Fig. 21 Recording the electrocardiogram of rat; a, typical trace; b, suitable positions for electrodes.

Table 24 Nutritional Requirement of Rat

A. General Requirements							
Age	**Specifi-cation**	**Body weig ht (kg)**	**Average Daily gain (gms)**	**Daily feed (gms)**	**Protein**		**DE/Kcal [MEMcal] ***
					Total (gms)	**Digestible (gms)**	
23 days	Growth	0.055	5.0	9	1.8	1.1	36
33 days	Growth	0.110	5.4	15	3.0	1.8	60
42 days	Growth	0.165	5.7	18	3.6	2.2	72
53 days	Growth	0.220	5.5	21	4.2	2.5	84
108 days	Growth	0.385	3.9	20	4.0	2.4	80
350 days adult	Mainte-nance	0.550	-	19	1.33	0.76	76
26 days	Growth	0.065	4.2	10	2.0	1.2	40
35 days	Growth	0.098	3.9	14	2.8	1.7	56
44 days	Growth	0.130	3.7	15	3.0	1.8	60
96 days	Growth	0.228	2.5	16	3.2	1.9	64
350 days adult	Mainte-nance	0.325	-	13	0.91	0.52	52
Adult	Pregnancy	-	4	19	3.8	2.3	76
	Lactation	-	0	33	6.6	4.0	131

*** Gross energy ; B. Vitamins**								
Age	**Specifi-cation**	**Ribo-flavin (mg)**	**Niacin (mg)**	**B_6 (mg)**	**Panto-thenic acid (mg)**	**B_{12} (μg)**	**A (IU)**	**D (IU)**
Adult	Growth	0.025* 0.25/ 100 gms diet	0.15* 1 5/ 100 gms diet	0.07 * 0.7/ 100 gms diet	0.08* 0.8/ 100 gms diet	0.05* 0.5/ 100 gms diet	20* 200/ 100 gms diet	10* 100/ 100 gms diet

Table 24 *Contd...*

Age	Specification	Riboflavin (mg)	Niacin (mg)	B_6 (mg)	Pantothenic acid (mg)	B_{12} (μg)	A (IU)	D (IU)
	Pregnancy	0.08* 0.4/ 100 gms diet	-	0.012* 0.6/ 100 gms diet	0.16* 0.08/ 100 gms diet	0.1* 0.5/ 100 gms diet	240* 1200/ 100 gms diet	0.6*3/ 100 gms diet
	Lactation	0.12* 0.4/ 100 gms diet	- -	0.012* 0.04/ 100 gms diet	0-3* 1.0/ 100 gms diet	0.15* 0.5/ 100 gms diet	360* 1200/ 100 gms diet	0 6* 2/100 gms 100 diet

C. Minerals						
Age	**Specification**	**Calcium (gms)**	**Iodine (gms)**	**Magnesium (gms)**	**Phosphorus (gms)**	**Sodium + Cholrine (gms)**
A	B	C	D	E	F	G
Adult	Growth	0.05* 0.5/ 100 gms diet	1.5 μg 15μg/ 100 gms diet	4 mg* 40 μg 100 gms diet	0.04* /100 gms diet	0.010 + 0.04 0.10/100 gms diet
	Gestation	0.12* 0.6/ 100 gms diet	3μg* 15 μg/ 100 gms diet	10mg* 50μg/ 100 gms. diet	0.10* 0.5/ 100 gms diet	0.015* 0.075/ 100 gms diet
	Lactation	0.18* 0.6/ 100gms diet	4.5 μg* 15μg/ 100gms. diet	0.15mg* 50μg/ 100gms. diet	0.15 μg* 0.5 μg/ 100 gm. diet	0.2 μg 0.68/ 100 gm μg diet

* Assuming a daily feed intake of 10 gms for growth, 20 gms for pregnancy, 30 gms for lactation.

Table 25 Parasitism in Rat

(A External Parasities)		
Species (Distribution) **A**	**Incidence in Laboratory** **B**	**Effect on Host** **C**
Acarina		
N-muris (Probably (Worldwide)	Common in some colonies, absent in others.	Wartlike, horny excrescences especially on ears.
Ornithonyssus bocoti (Worldwide)	Rate in some colonies, common in others.	Debility, anemia, decreased reproduction death.
R. ensifera (worldwide)	Common	Self-inflicted dermal trauma
Siphonaptera		
A	**B**	**C**
Nosopsyllus fasciatus (Worldwide)	Rare	Acts as intermediate host for *Hymenolepis diminuta & H. nana.*
Xenopsylla cheopis (Worldwide)	Uncommon	Act as intermediate host for *Hymenolepis diminuta & H. nana.*
Mallophage & Anoplura		
P. spinulosa (Worldwide)	Common in some colonies, rare or absent in othets	Pruritus, anemia, vector of *Rickettsia typhi & Haemobartonella muris*

(B. Internal Parasites)			
Species (Distribution) **A**	**Incidence in Laboratory** **B**	**Host (Localization)** **C**	**Effects on Host** **D**
Nematoda			
Syphaciamuris (Worldwide)	Common	Caecum-colon	Apparently nonpathogenic except in heavy infections.
Platyhelminthes-Cestoda			
Hymenolepis diminuta	Uncommon	Intestine	Usually inapparent ; sometimes enteritis.
H. nana (Worldwide)	Common	Intestine	Retarded growth, weight loss
T. taeniaeformis (Worldwide)	Common in some colonies, absent in others	Rat Liver	Hepatic cyst formation ; sometimes hepatic sarcoma.

Table 25 *Contd...*

Protozoa			
Species (Distribution) **A**	**Incidence in Laboratory** **B**	**Host (Localization)** **C**	**Effects on Host** **D**
Toxoplasma gondii (Worldwide)	Common in some colonies ; uncommon or absent in others.	Rat Various tissues	Inapparent to fatal disease with varied signs
(C. Viral Diseases)			
Virus Group [Examples]	**Morphology [Nucleic Acid]**	**Host [Natural Transmission**	**Remarks**
Tacaribe -LCM viruses [Limphocytic choriomeningitis ; viruses causing South American hemorrhagic fevers]	Similar to gaviruses but larger up to 110 nm [Single stranded RNA]	Rat [Arthropod vectors ; in feces & urine]	Virion contains granules similar to ribosomes.

(D. Rickettsial Parasdites)		
Species	**Disease or Disorder**	**Method of Transmission**
Haemobartonella spp.	Haemobartonellosis, anemia	Flea to host
R. Sibirica	Siberian tick typhus	Tick to host
R. tsutsugamushi	Tsutsugamushi fever (Scrub typhus)	Mite to host
R. typhi	Murine or endemic typhus	Flea faeces

Table 26 Chemical Composition and Physical Properties of Lymph of Rat

Conditions	Source of Lymph	Constituent	Value	
			Lymph	Plasma or serum
A	B	C	D	E
Fasted, anaesthetized	Thoracic duct	Calcium, meq/1tr.	5.9	7.4
		Calcium, meq/1tr.	5.4 ± 0.3	5.6 ± 0.2
		Chloride, meq/1tr,	103 ± 2	101 ± 2

Table 26 *Contd...*

Conditions A	Source of Lymph B	Constituent C	Value	
			Lymph D	Plasma or serum E
		Magnesium, meq/1tr.	1.7 ± 0.1	1.7 ± 0.1
		Potassium, meq/1tr.	5.1	4.9
		Potassium, meq/1tr	5.2 ± 0.2	5.4 ± 0.2
		Sodium, meq/1tr.	158	151
		Sodium, meq/1tr.	145 ± 2	145 ± 1
		Fatty acids, meq/1tr.	9.6	10.4
		Fatty acids, mg/100ml.	(742-1460)	N.A
		Fatty acids, free, mg/ 100 ml	39.9	23.1
		Fatty acids, esterified, eq/kl	11.75 ± 1.24	N. A.
		Triglycerides, mg/100 ml	273.2	74.3
		Phopholipid, mg/100 ml	203	138
		Phospholipid, mg/100 ml	86.5	70.6
		Cholesterol, total, mg/ 100 ml	(2.3-62.4)	N. A.
		Cholesterol, total mg/ 100 ml	72	51
		Cholesterol, total mg/ 100 ml.	3 ± 5.3	50 ± 10.5
		Cholesterol, free, mg/ 100 ml	9.2 ± 1.5	8.2 ± 1.7
		Cholesterol esters mg/ 100 ml	28.7 ± 4.5	41.8 ± 9.5

Table 26 *Contd...*

Conditions	Source of Lymph	Constituent	Value	
			Lymph	Plasma or serum
A	B	C	D	E
Fed	*Lymphatics Hepatic*	Total lipid, mg/100 ml	240(148-399)	267(202-290)
		Cholate, mg/100 ml	1.5 (0.7-1.9)	2.6 (2.4-3.0)
		Cholesterol. total, mg/100 ml	33 (12-28)	65 (52-71)
		Cholesterol, total, mg/100 ml	36.0 ± 4.2	47.7 ± 2.8
	Intestinal	Total lipid, mg/ 100 ml	1150	220
Fasted		Total lipid, mg/100 ml	1590	378
		Fatty acids, mg/100 ml	(1000-1572)	N. A.
		Cholesterol, total mg/100 ml	55.2 ± 6.2	47.7 ± 2.8
		Cholesterol, total, mg/100ml	(62.1-69.2)	N. A.
Fed		Cholesterol, free, mg/100ml	27	17
Fasted		Cholesterol, free, mg/100ml	34	24
Fed		Cholesterol esters, mg/ 100 ml	86	41
Fasted		Cholesterol esters, mg/ 100 ml	120	49
		Fatty acids in triglycerides,% Palmitic (16:0)	20.4	23.5
		Stearic (18 : 0)	26.6	27.7
		Oleic (18 : 1)	33.3	27.2
		Linoleic(18: 2)	5.8	5.1
		Octadecatrienoic (18 : 3)	1.8	2.8

Table 26 *Contd...*

Conditions	Source of Lymph	Constituent	Value	
			Lymph	Plasma or serum
A	B	C	D	E
		Fatty acids in phospholipid, % Palmitic (16: 0)	28.9	22.3
		Stearic (18:0)	25.6	25.6
		Oleic (18.1)	23.1	22.3
		Linoleic (18:2)	8.6	14.9
		Octadecatri-enoic (18 : 3)	1.5	3.4
		Fatty acids in cholesterol esters, % Palmitic (16:0)	16.1	17.6
		Oleic (18:1)	38.5	37.9
		Linoleic (18 : 2)	23.2	24.9
		Octadecatri-enoic (18 : 3)	2.6	3.2
		Triglycerides, mg/100 ml.	14	76
		Phospholipid, mg/100 ml.	19	119
		Phospholipid mg/100 ml	44.6(39.5-54.1)	119.3 (108.5-144.1)
		Cholesterol, total mg/100 ml	2.3(17.3-32.0)	88.9 (55.6-112.1)
		Cholesterol free + esters, mg/100 ml.	27	134
		Carbohydrates & related compound		
Thoracic duct		Fucose, mg/100 ml.	5.9	
		Glucose, mg/100 ml.	121	105

Table 26 *Contd...*

Conditions	Source of Lymph	Constituent	Value	
			Lymph	Plasma or serum
A	B	C	D	E
		γ-Glucose, mg/100 ml	209 (200-220)	192 (165-230)
		γ-Globulin, g/100 ml.	0.26 ± 0.01	0.71 ± 0.03
		γ-Globulin, g/100 ml	3.40 ± 0.07	1.14 ± 0.24
		γ-Globulin, g/100 ml	0.40 ± 0.09	1.37 ± 0.17
		γ-Globulin, g/100 ml	0.43 ± 0.08	1.61 ± 0.08
		γ-Globulin, g/100 ml	0.47 ± 0.06	1.28 ± 0.17
		Protein, total g/100 ml.	1.91	5.68
Fasted, anaesthetized		Protein, total g/100 ml.	3.06 (1.64-4.48)	5.82 (4.40-7.24)
		Protein, total, g/100 ml.	4.1	5.7
		Protein, total, g/100 ml.	4.18	–
		Protein, total, g/100 ml.	3.94 ± 0.16	5.69 ± 0.11
		Albumin, g/100 ml.	1.29	3.20
		Globulin, g/100 ml.	2.15	3.31
		α-Globulin, g/100 ml.	0.68 ± 0.03	1.44 ± 0.04
		α_1–Globulin, g/100ml.	0.46	0.85
		α_2–Globulin, g/100 ml.	0.20	0.32
		γ– Globulin, g/100 ml.	0.44 ± 0.22	0.42 ± 0.05
		Amino acids, mg/100 ml.		
		Alanine	2.0	3.8

Table 26 *Contd...*

Conditions A	Source of Lymph B	Constituent C	Value: Lymph D	Value: Plasma or serum E
		Arginine	1.3	1.8
		Aspartic-acid	Trace	0.2
		Cysteine + cystine	Trace	Trace
		Glutamic acid	0.7	1.1
Thoracic duct		Glycine	2.1	2.7
		Histidine	1.2	1.3
		Isoleucine	1.4	1.2
		Leucine	2.2	2.0
		Lysine	4.2	4.8
		Methionine	0.5	0.8
		Phenylalanine	1.1	1.1
		Proline	1.1	1.5
		Tarrine	1.5	3.8
		Threonine	1.7	2.4
		Tyrosine	0.9	1.3
		Valine	2.1	2.1
		Purine derivatives, mg/100 ml		
		Adenine + Uracil	0.223 (0.205-0.230)	–
		Cytosine	0.230 (0.200-0.260)	-
		Guanine	0.127 (0.100-0.140)	-
		Uric acid	0.416 (0.371-0.520)	-

Table 27 Tissue Growth and Renewal in Rat

Organ A	Growth Specification B	Age/other Specification C	Tissue Growth & Renewal characteristics* D
Nervous system			
Cerebellum	Proliferation	> 3 wk old	Proliferative external granular layer present from which basket cells are formed

Table 27 *Contd...*

Digestive System			
Alimentary canal : Buccail mucosa	Replacement	N. S.	T_t = 4.3 da, 16-24 da.
Gingivae	Replacement	N. S.	Epithelium : T_t = 10-44 da
Lips	Replacement	N. S.	Epithelium : T_t = 15 da.
Tongue	Proliferation	Embryo	Epithelium : T_c = 23 hrs T_s = 5.6 hr.
	Replacement	N. S.	Epithelium : T_t of dorsal surface = 4.9 da . T_t of ventral surface = 7.7 da.
Esophagus	Proliferation	N. S.	T_s = 5-10 hr ; Basal layer: LI = 20.0 %
	Replacement	N. S.	T_t = 9-12 da.
	Regenerative Capacity	N. S.	Re- epitheliazation occurs.
Stomach	Proliferation	N. S.	MI affected by stress
	Regeneration Capacity	N. S.	Migration occurs with 24 hr of induction of ulcer.
Neck	Replacement	N. S.	Mucous cells ; T_t = 6.5 da.
Body	Replacement	N. S.	Surface cells : T_t = 30 da. Gland cells. T_t = 1.8 da.
Pylorus	Replacement	N. S.	Surface cells : T_t = 1.9 da.
Duodenum	Proliferation	N. S.	Increase in cell number affected hormones, especially thyroid hormone. Enzyme activity increase as cells migrate up villi.
	Proliferation	Weaning 54 & 147 da old	MI = 3.4%T_c = 10-11 hr ; T_s = 7 hr; T_m = 0.7 hr.
		Adult	MI = 5.6%
	Life span & replacement	N. S.	T_t = 1.6 da
Jejunum	Proliferation	N. S.	$T_c \approx 11$ hr; T_m = 1 hr. T_s = 6.5 – 7.5 hr. No. of proliferative cells increase during lactation.
	Life span & replacement	N. S.	T_t = 1.3 da

Table 27 *Contd...*

Organ	Growth Specification	Age/other Specification	Tissue Growth & Renewal Characteristics*
A	B	C	D
Ileum	Proliferation	N. S.	T_s = 7.6 hr.
	Life span & replacement	N. S.	T_t = 1.4 – 2.6 da.
Total small intestine	Replacement	Weaning	Cell replacement rate = 112 × 10^6/ da
		Young	Cell replacement rate = 914 × 10^6/ da
		Adult	Cell replacement rate = 1795 × 10^6 / da
	Regenerative capacity	N. S.	Mucosal wounds are repaired at all levels by epithelial migration & proliferation.
Colon	Proliferation	N. S.	T_s = 8 hr.
	Life span & replacement	N. S.	T_t = 10 da
	Regeneration capacity	N. S.	Mucosal repair & new gland formation occur ; variations are due to amount of granulation tissue.
Accessory organs of digestion	Proliferation	N. S.	Acinar cells : LI = 0.4 – 1.0%, increases to ≈24% 2 da after isoproterenol is given
Salivary glands		15-da embryo	Duct cells : LI = 3% 28.Interstitial cells : LI = 0.6% T_c – 16hr. T_s – 6 hr.
		18-da embryo	T_c = 24 hr ; T_z = 5 hr.
	Replacement	N. S.	Acinar & tubular cells divide.
	Regenerative capacity	N. S.	Slight regeneration by proliferation of ancinar cells & intercalated ducts. Regeneration by acinar cell division in 1st week, followed by proliferation of ducts and formation of acini form terminal portions.

Table 27 *Contd...*

Organ	Growth Specification	Age/other Specification	Tissue Growth & Renewal Characteristics*
A	**B**	**C**	**D**
Parotid	Proliferation	N. S.	Acinar cells: mitosis / 1000 = 1.02 $\pm$ 0.23; MI = 0.102 $\pm$ 0.023%
	Life span	N. S.	Acinar cells : 41 da 93
Sublingual	Proliferation	N. S.	Acinar cells : mitosis / 1000 = 0.70 $\pm$ 0.23 ; MI = 0.07 $\pm$ 0.023%
	Life span	N. S.	Acinar cells ; 60 da.
Submandibular	Proliferation	N. S.	Acinar cells ; $\pm$ mitosis/ 1000 = 0.64 $\pm$ 0.17
			Tubular cells ; mitosis / 1000 = 0.44 $\pm$ 0.12 ; MI = 0.044 $\pm$ 0.012%
	Life span	N. S.	Acinar cells : 65 da. Tabular cells : 95 da.
Liver	Proliferation	N. S.	Littoral cells : LI = 0.8 –2.3%
		1 da old	T_c = 14 hr ; T_s = 7 hr ; T_m = 0.3 hr.
		3 wk old	T_c = 22 hr ; T_s = 9 hr; T_m = 1.7 hr.
		5 wk old	T_c = 21 hr ; T_s = 9 hr ; T_m = 1.0 hr.
		8 wk old	T_c = 48 hr ; T_s = 16 hr ; T_m = 1.7 hr.
		Adult	Proliferation shows diurnal rhythm. T_s = 18 hr. LI = 1.0% MI = 0.0001– 0.0005% After partial hepatectomy ; T_c = 16.5-24 hr ; $T_s \approx$ 80 hr ; T_m = 1.0 hr.
	Mode of growth	N. S.	In early life, by cell division ; in later life, by increased cell size. Cell size increases greatly between 7-34 da, increases slightly more by 95 da. Ploidy increases with age.
		7 da	No. of nuclei in liver = 228 × 10^6.

Table 27 *Contd...*

Organ	Growth Specification	Age/other Specification	Tissue Growth & Renewal Characteristics*
A	B	C	D
		17 da	No. of nuclei in liver = 687 × 10^6.
		35 da	No. of nuclei in liver = 1310 × 10^6.
		95 da	No. of nuclei in liver = 2655 × 10^6.
	Life span	N.S.	Form 190 da to death
	Regenerative capacity	N. S.	Can occur repeatedly. Normal weight almost regained 3 wk after two-thirds hepatectomy ; major regrowth in 7 da. Regeneration response occurs after 10-30% of liver is resected. Age affects regenerative capacity.
Pancrease	Proliferation	embryo	T_c = ;0 hr ; T_8 = 6 hr.
		adult	Acinar cells : LI = 0.46%; duct cells : LI = 0.8% ; interstitial cells : LI = 0.06%.
	Regenerative capacity	N. S.	Slow regeneration rate ; LI is 3 times greater after partial pancreatectomy, and 20 times greater after administration of ethionine.
Circulatory System			
Heart	Mode of growth	birth -22 da	Cell division
		birth-4 mo	LI decreases to a minimum
		48 da	No increase in cell nuclei
	Replacement	N. S.	No
	Regenerative capacity	N. S.	Probably negligible ; hypertrophy caused by increased fiber size.
			In compensatory hypertrophy, LI of connective tissue & endothelial cells rises to 1-2%

Table 27 *Contd...*

Organ	Growth Specification	Age/other Specification	Tissue Growth & Renewal Characteristics*
A	B	C	D
Blood Erythrocytes & Precursors	Proliferation	N. S.	Erythroblasts : $T_c = 9.16$ hr ; $T_s = 5 - 8$ hr ; $T_m \approx 0.5$ hr. LI = 30 – 70%. Stem cells : T_c = 23-35 hr.
	Mode of growth	N. S.	When cell growth stops. RNA & protein synthesis decrease and hemoglobin synthesis increases.
	Life span	N. S.	45-68 da.
	Replacement	N. S.	2.4×10^7 cells/hr enter circulation.
	Regeneration capacity	N. S.	Recovery in 7da from 30% blood loss. During protracted anemia,cell cycle shortens and production may increase to 5 times normal.
Granulocytes & precursors	Proliferation	N. S.	Monocytes : $T_c = 21$ hr ; $T_s = 12.5$ hr.
	Life span & replacement	N. S.	Moncytes :half time for disappearance from blood = 3.1 da.
Lymphocytes	Proliferation	N. S.	84×10^6 cells / hr are exchanged between spleen and blood. T_c = 6-8 hr.
		100 g	Small lymphocytes : total no. = 1150×10^6; no. in spleen = 2.0×10^6 / mg; no. in thymus = 3.5×10^6 / mg.
		40-60 da old	Maximum weight attained in thymus.
		65 da old	Maximum weight attained in mesenteric lymph nodes.
		100 da old	Maximum weight attained in spleen and cervical nodes.

Table 27 *Contd...*

Organ	Growth Specification	Age/other Specification	Tissue Growth & Renewal Characteristics*
A	B	C	D
		N. S.	Precursors to antibody-forming cells. Peak LI = 4-6.5% on 6th day of secondary response.
	Life Span	N. S.	Wide variation in life Bone marrow lymphocytes are probably short-lived, and one-third of the blood lymphocytes short-lived. Long –lived lymphocytes recirculate from lymph to blood, and have potential for division & immunological competence
		N. S.	Small lymphocytes : 14 da to 9 mo.
	Replacement	N. S.	Thoracic duct : $(30 - 60) \times 10^6$ cells/hr. Thymus : $T_t \approx 60$ hr. Thymus can produce no. equal to total lymphocytes in body in 2-3 da.
		N. S.	20×10^6 cells (1.7%) replaced/hr.
Platelets	Production	N. S.	Maturation occurs from stem cell → polyploid precursor cell → megakaryoblast (Stage I) → promegakaryocyte (Stage II) Platelets are then formed by fragmentation of granular megakaryocyte cytoplasm (Stage III).

Table 27 *Contd...*

Organ	Growth Specification	Age/other Specification	Tissue Growth & Renewal Characteristics*
A	B	C	D
	Cell division	N. S.	Rare in megakaryocytes C mitosis and multipolar mitosis without cytokinesis observed in ≈0.8% megakaryocytes. Endoreduplication cycle in ≈9 % lasting 9 hr ; T_s = 8 hr; LI = 7.3%.
	Life span	N. S.	4 – 5 da
Lymphatic System			
Thymus	Mode of growth	N. S.	No. of nuclei increases rapidly to 48 da old, then decreases
Urogenital System			
Kidney	Proliferation	N.S.	Tubular epithelium : T_s = 7 hr; LI = 0.54 ± 0.02% ; MI = 0.023 ± 0.01%
	Mode of growth	N. S.	Increased no. and size of cells and structure mainly by hypertrophy in mature subjects.
		N. S.	No. of cells increases rapidly in early life.
		Birth-2wk old	No. of nephrons doubles.
		7-90 da old	No. of nuclei increase 6.5 times original no.
		17-34 da old	Size of proximal convoluted tubule cells increases.
	Life span	N. S.	Majority of cells survive throughout life
	Regenerative capacity	N. S.	Increased proliferation after unilateral nephrectomy and ligation of ureter. Tubular cells hy pertrophy with increased demand.

Table 27 *Contd...*

Organ	Growth Specification	Age/other Specification	Tissue Growth & Renewal Characteristics*
A	B	C	D
Bladder	Proliferation	N. S.	Transitional epithelium; $T_t = 33$ da * , 64 da^+
Ureter	Proliferation	N.S.	Transitional epithelium: $T_t = 49$ da.
* Superficial cells. + Deep cells			
Bladder & Ureter	Replacement	N. S.	Transitional epithelium cells move from deep to superficial layer over a period of weeks.
Testis	Duration of spermatogenesis	N. S.	16 -48 ; 4 cycles of the seminiferous epithelium are required for complete spermatogenesis ; average length of spermatogenic wave = 25-28 mm. Transport of spermatozoa along epididymis and vas deferens last 12 da.
Spermatogonia	Regenerative capacity	N. S.	Regeneration after injury occurs if spermatogonia type A survive.
Type A_I	Proliferation	N. S.	$T_c \approx 144$ hr ; $T_s = 19.5$ hr.
Type AII	Proliferation	N. S.	$T_c = 39$ hr ; $T_s = 20.5$ hr.
Type AIII	Proliferation	N.S.	$T_c = 42$ hr ; $T_s = 21.0$ hr.
Type AIV	Proliferation	N.S.	$T_c = 42$ hr ; $T_s = 23.0$ hr.
Intermediate	Proliferation	N. S.	$T_c = 42$ hr ; $T_s = 24.0$ hr.
Type B	Proliferation	N. S.	$T_c = 42$ hr ; $T_s = 25.5$ hr
Prostategland	Proliferation	Birth –20 da old	Mitoses numerous
		100 da old	Mitoses few

Table 27 *Contd...*

Organ	Growth Specification	Age/other Specification	Tissue Growth & Renewal Characteristics*
A	B	C	D
	Mode of growth	N. S.	Hypertrophy and hyperplasia very greatly.
		N. S.	Growth affected by hormonal activity.
		Birth – 20 da old	Cell proliferation.
		11-55	Cell height increases from 18 μ to 34 μ ; acinus diameter increases from 43 μ to 170 μ.
Ovary	Regenerative capacity	N. S.	Regenerative activity of germinal epithelium after horomone stimulation
Follicles	Proliferation	N. S.	Granulosa cells T_s = 8 hr.
Graafian	Proliferation	N.S.	Granulosa cell proliferate.
Oocytes	Proliferation	N. S.	Occurs in fetal period. Total no. of oocytes is related to age: log (no.) = 4.561 – 0. 476 log (age in days).
	Regenerative	N. S.	No regeneration.
Cervix	Proliferation and mode of growth	N. S.	T_t = 5.5 da. Surface epithelium : T_t = 5.9 da. Grandular epithelium : T_t = 10. da ; MI = 0.079 ± 0.05%. Lumen epithelium : MI = 0.94 ± 5%. Connective tissue : MI = 0.07% circular muscle : MI = 0.1%. longitudinal muscle : MI = 0.02%
		Diestrus	Epithelium : T_c ≈ 33 hr ; T_s = 5-6 hr; LI ≈ 17%; MI = 2.4%. Stroma : T_c is very long ; T_s = 7 hr; LI = 0.45%.

Table 27 *Contd...*

Organ	Growth Specification	Age/other Specification	Tissue Growth & Renewal Characteristics*
A	B	C	D
		Pseudogestation	Epithelium : LI = 2%
		2nd da	Stroma : LI = 4%
		4th da	Epithelium : LI = 0% Stroma : LI = 11%.
		5th & 6th da Mechanical Distension of cervix After 1 da	Epithelium : LI = 16% Glandular epithelium : MI = 0.1 ± 0.08%. Lumen epithelium : MI = 2.1 ± 0.06%. connective tissue : MI = 0.6 ± 0.2%.
		After 2 da	Circular muscle : MI = 1.7 ± 1.6%. longitudinal muscle : MI = 0.19 ± 0.03%.
Vagina		After estrogen	LI increases with increasing estrogen doses & shortening of cell cycle.
Muscular System			
Smooth muscle	Mode of growth	Adult during hypertension	Increased no. of arterial & arteriolar muscle cells.
	Regenerative capacity	N. S.	Limited regeneration after injury, fibrous scar usual. In gut hypertrophy & some proliferative activity occur.
Striated muscle	Proliferation	14-da embryo	LI = 34%
		21-da embryo	LI = 1.5%
	Mode of growth	During development	Cell division
		adult	Hypertrophy
		N. S.	No. of nuclei increases with age.
		Suckling to 79-94 old	Muscle fiber no. remains constant muscle weight increases 9-21 times the original.

Table 27 *Contd...*

Organ	Growth Specification	Age/other Specification	Tissue Growth & Renewal Characteristics*
A	B	C	D
	Replacement	N. S.	Little or none.
Gastrocnemius	Mode of growth	17-95 da old	No. of nuclei increases 3.8 times the original, and fiber size 5.5 times.
Tibialis anterior	Mode of growth	Young	1.21-1.75% of nuclei enter mitosis every 24 hr.
Integumentary System			
Skin	Proliferation	N. S.	LI = 2.9 ± 0.2%. MI : 1-2% : varies with age.
	Replacement	N. S.	Adjustment between cell loss & cell formation. Differentiated cells remain in basal layer before moving to superficial layers.
	Regenerative capacity	N. S.	Re – epithelialization of wounds by proliferation & migration of cells, amount of proliferation depends on size of would. Regeneration possible from hair follicles. Growth granulation tissue checked by epithelium overgrowth.
Abdominal wall	Life span	N. S.	19.4 da
Ear	Life span	N. S.	34.5 da
Sole of foot	Life span	N. S.	19.1 da. Basal layer : 16.9 da. Stratum granulosum : 2.2 da
Skin out-growths : Hair	Growth rate	N. S.	> 1.2 mm/da

Table 27 *Contd...*

Organ	Growth Specification	Age/other Specification	Tissue Growth & Renewal Characteristics*
A	B	C	D
	Hair cycle	N. S.	Waves of hair growth sweep posteriorly and dorsally, become less frequent with age. Follicle : growth phase = 17-19 da
Nails	Growth rate	29-683 da old	0.0056-0.0109 cm/da
Endocrine Glands			
Hypophysis	Proliferation	N. S.	In light : dark cycle of 12 : 12 hr. LI = 0.51 $\pm$ 0.04%. In light : dark cycle of 24 0 hr : LI = 0.32 $\pm$ 0.02%, % acidophils increased from 13.7% to 24.2% of total no.
		Castrate	In light : dark cycle of 12 : 12 hr : LI = 0.90 $\pm$ 0.09%
		2wk later	Increased LI is 3-6 times higher than control value of $\approx$ 0.08.
		Female	LI is higher than in male
		Diestrus	34-39 labeled cells/mm^2
		Estrus	299 $\pm$ 18.9 labeled cells/mm^2
Anterior lobe, lateral area	Proliferation	57 g 349 g	LI = 0.63 $\pm$ 0.06% LI = 0.18 $\pm$ 0.06%
Medial area	Proliferation	57 g 349 g	LI = 0.44 $\pm$ 0.07% LI = 0.17 $\pm$ 0.04%
Intermediate lobe	Proliferation	57 g 349 g	LI = 0 63% LI = 0.01%
Posterior lobe	Proliferation	57 g 349 g	LI = 0.33% LI = 0.39%
Suprarenal gland	Proliferation	Young adult	MI is higher than for adult MI = 0.12%.
Cortex	Proliferation	185 g	LI = 0.15 %, MI = 0.006%.
	Life span	N. S.	Uncertain

Table 27 *Contd...*

Organ	Growth Specification	Age/other Specification	Tissue Growth & Renewal Characteristics*
A	B	C	D
	Replacement	N. S.	Cell division & migration of cells from superficial to deeper layers. Labeling experiment have not always shown migration in unstressed animals.
	Regenerative capacity	N. S.	Repair by cell division after damage, limited repair adult.
Zona glomerulosa	Proliferation	6 da old	T $\approx$80 hr, longer in inner zones T_s $\approx$ 8 hr. LI – 10.9%.
		185 g	Labeled cells : LI increased after castration.
		Adult	MI = 0.17%
Zona fasciculata	Proliferation	6 da old	LI = 2.6%, 0.3%
		185 g	Labeled cells : MI = 47.6%
Zona fasciculata & Zona capsula	Proliferation	Adult	MI = 0.13%
Zona reticularis	Proliferation	6 da old	LI = 0%
		185 g	Labeled cells : MI = 41.3%
		Adult	MI = 0.6%
	Life span	N. S.	Phagocytosis occurs
Transition zone	Proliferation	6 da old	LI = 9.1%
Medulla	Mode of growth	N. S.	Postnatal growth by hypertrophy
Thyroid gland	Proliferation	N. S.	Follicular cells : < 1-9 mitoses/10,000 cells. Stromal cells : <1- 4 mitosis/10,000 cells.
		2-4 wk old	LI $\approx$3%
		6-8 wk old	LI = 0.3%
	Regenerative		Hypertrophy of remaining gland after partial thyroidectomy
	Capacity	Rat	Follicular & stromal cells: proliferation occurs with prophylthiouracil treatment.

Based on Biological Data Book.

SECTION-B

EXPERIMENTS ON MICE AND RATS

This section of the book compiles some experiments on mice and rats for screening the pharmacologically active substances.

Albino swiss mice are smallest laboratory animals and are considered as the most widely used laboratory animals. This animal can be breed uniformly, is cheap and easy to handle and being tiny are sensitive to little doses of test substances.

Mice are widely used in screening of chemotherapeutic agents. On the other hand albino rats are one of the commonest laboratory animals. Its popularity as laboratory animal is next only to that of mice. The laboratory rats can be breed to obtain pure and uniform strains and is found to be very sturdy to withstand long period of experimentation under anaesthesia. They are also widely used like mice for screening of chemotherapeutic agents.

Here, two types of experiments have been discussed. One is intact preparation and another is isolated preparation of two rodents. There are big differences between the two types of experiment.

The effects of a drug in a whole animal (intact preparation) are complicated by the possibility that what is observed is the consequence of the drug acting at many sites at once.

The effects of the drug observed will depend upon the rate of excretion and metabolism and may be quite different from those observed with isolated preparation, where the drug is added in a known concentration at a known time to small piece of tissue and washed out at a known time. Intact preparations have the great advantage that they indicate the likely clinical effects of a drug much better than isolated preparations but they have the disadvantage to the effect that it may be much more difficult, to work out how the drug is acting. In fact, both types of experiments are necessary.

EXPERIMENT 1

Behavioural Test in Mice

A battery of tests has been designed which permits a series of suppositions based on them, so that under certain results neuroleptic activity may be anticipated. No single activity is specific for the neuroleptic property. Those substances which depress CNS, Come to light in various ways. There are some ataractic agents that cruse no clear loss of alertness but these type of agents potentiate the activity of other CNS depressants. The degree and nature of CNS depression action varies according to the affected area of nervous system.

Six types of experimental tests constitute the battery of tests. The investigator will examine the results of blind screening in the event of it being performed before commencing the present battery of tests, as there are some duplications. If the test compounds that he has to screen were not found by a preliminary blind screening, he may proceed to perform the neuroharmacological part of the blind screening first.

Material and Equipment

Jingle cage, Rotating rod, Metallic wire, Rectangular box, Pyrex-glass tube, Bell-Jar, Electronic thermometer, Na - pentobarbitone, Morphine, Iminodipropionitrile, trans-cinnamyl carbarmate, strychnine, pentylylenetetrazol, Ataractic agent.

Procedure

1. ***Behaviour***

   Tranquillizers usually effect a state of sedation or indifference in mice, expecially when applied at the higher doses. No attempt is made to quantify the observations, which nevertheless from a part of the screening programms. The presence or absence of sedation in mice given the test substances is noted.

2. ***Motility***

   (a) *Jingle-Cage*

   Rats are injected with the test substance. Their motions are registered with the aid of a "Jingle-cage" after 1 minute and after 30 minutes, for a period of 10 minutes. The Jingle cage is a cage mounted on springs or bearings so that all but the slightest movements of the animal makes the cage to swing to and fro slightly and thus to close the electrical circuit of a counter. The number of movements of the animal during a period is thus recorded.

(b) *Rotating Rod*

Mice are placed on a surface-rubbed rod of wood, 2 cm, in diameter, turning at the rate of 10 rotations per minute. Circular sections divide the linear space of the rod into 10 lengths, so that 10 mice are tested together. The control mouse is able to stand on the rod for longer than 300 seconds. The treated mice are placed on the rod at intervals, and the time of the fa1l from the rod is noted. The test is terminated at 300 seconds. From the number of mice in a group that fall from the rod before 300 seconds, the ED50 may be calculated for any given interval after administration of the test substance.

Male and female mice are used, Untreated animals are placed on a horizontal rotating, wooden rod having a diameter of 32 mm, and rotating at the rate of 5 revolutions per minute, Animals that rest on the rod for 3 or more minutes in two successive trials are selected and placed in groups of five. Each group is then injected **s.** c. with a drug and placed on the rod at intervals of 30, 60, 90, 120 and 150 minutes. after dosage. If an animal fails more than once to remain on the rod for 3 minutes., the test is considered positive, that is, motor incoordination is present.

(c) *Traction Test*

By means of four paws mice are suspended to a metallic wire, stretched horizontally. The normal mouse effects a better posture in less than 5 seconds. The number of animals is noted who are not able to touch the wire with at least one of the hind-paws. The ED50 is computed in the usual way : the dose inhibiting 50% of the animals from touching the wire with a hind paw, within 5 seconds after placement on the wire, and 30 minutes. following injection of a drug.

(d) *Evasion*

This is a test of the residual curiosity of the mouse. Ten mice of group are placed in rectangular box having an inclined place by which the mice can escape. The number of mice remaining in the box after 5 minutes, is noted. The ED50 is the dose inhibiting the escape of 50% of the mice at a given time after injection.

(e) *Chimney Test*

Pyrex-glass tubes, 30 cm. long, are used. The internal diameter varies with the animal's weight : for mice weighing 16 to 18 gms. the diameter is 22 mm ; for mice weighing 18 to 20 gm, 25 mm ; for mice weighing 20 to 22 gms, 28 mm. Each tube has a mark 20 cm. from its base. At the end of the tube near the mark, a mouse is introduced. When the animal reaches the other en of the tube, towards which it is pushed if necessary with a rod, the tube is moved to the vertical position. Immediately, the mouse makes effort to climb the tube backwards. The test is positive when the mouse reaches the mark in less than 30 seconds. Untreated mice reach the mark almost always within this interval. For each does, groups of 6 to 10 mice are used. The ED50, defined as the dose necessary to lower the number of positively performing mice to 50% is calculated for specified times after administration, of the test substance. The mice are sometimes used again, as there was no havituation of them.

3. *Potentiation of Depressants*

(a) *Barbiturate*

The test substance is given 30 minutes or longer before pentobarbitone, 30 mg/kg, i.p. The number of animals exhibiting ataxia, anesthesia, and sedation is recorded every 5 minutes up to 60 minutes.

When the animals have recovered completely from the Na-pentobarbitone, an i.p, ED50 dose of an ataractic agent may prevail on a second, prolonged hypnosis.

(b) *Potentiation of Ethar*

Under a glass bell-jar, 10 ml. of ether is introduced at the rate of 1 ml. per minute. Control mice, placed in the container just before the commencement of the influx, are all anaesthetized within 7 minutes, following the end of the influx. The animal, then left in the open air, regains the righting reflex in 2 minutes, and 24 seconds, (mean time). Ataractic agents lessen the time for the induction of anaesthesia and prolong the time from the placement of the mouse in the air until the appearance of the righting reaction.

(c) *Potentiation of Morphine*

This is a hot-plate test. The hot-plate is kept 57°, and the time until the licking of the paw is noted.

4. ***Central Psychosedation Other Seizures***

When iminodipropionitrile is given to mice, a characteristic seizure follows : the mice move in circles and shake their heads in a motion. Ataractic agents may antagonize the syndrome. A similar seizure, likewise antagonised, is caused by trans cinnamyl carbamate.

5. ***Anticonvulsive Tests***

Antagonism toward strychnine and pentylenetetrazol convulsions are tested by the method of intraveneous perfusion. The value of these tests is subject to question in relation to tranquillizers.

6. ***Hypothermia***

The sigmoidal temperature of mice is recorded every 1/2 hr. Groups of 6 mice are used for each dose. The temperature of the control mice is 37.0°C to 38.2°C during 6 hours. Ataractic agents cause the temperature to fall as the dose is increased, even so low as 28.6°C. The animals are kept in a room at 25°C.

EXPERIMENT 2

Test of Ataractic Agents by Electrical Stimulation of Pairs of Mice

Although the conditioned avoidance response has been a advantageous method for screening ataractic agents, the behaviour of selected, arrogant mice with fighting character is considered a more sensitive index to evalute the tranquillizing property than the conditioned avoidance response.

Material and Equipment

Parallel copper rods (4.77 mm. in diameter and fixed 6.35 mm. apart), Bell-Jar, D.C. Electric shock machine (60 V), Test drug.

Procedure

1. Pairs of mice (20 - 30 gms.) are placed on parallel copper rods and after a bell-jar is placed over the mice, they are given feeble electric shocks from shock giving mechine.
2. The machine will provide pulses of direct current, 0.5 msec. in duration, at the rate of 20 shocks/sec.
3. At least ½ of the pairs show 2-3 fighting responses in 1 minute.
4. Those pairs that show the response are retained for further use in individual cages. They are given test drug 30 minutes. Before testing them for the fighting response.
5. Pairs of mice that do not fight once in 1 minute. on the rods are scored as having no response.
6. ED50, that is the dose necessary for elimination of the fighting response in 50% of the pairs can be computed with groups of pairs administered with appropriate doses.

EXPERIMENT 3

Test of Analgesic Agents in Mice

Stimuli (Physical, thermal or Chemical) are employed in mice to evaluate analgesic property of compound (either synthetic or natural). To eschew false positive result, a discoordination test is carried out in animal by rotaing drum method.

A. Material and Equipment

Artery clip, Analgesic test substance.

Procedure

1. Selection made from two groups of mice: one group is considered as control and another group as treated (which are treated with analgesic substance).
2. Artery clip with thin rubber sleeves is applied to the base of tail of both group of mice for 30 seconds. Control mice make continuous endeavours to farce out the clip by means of biting it. The pressure exerted by the clip is so adjusted that it is just sufficient to make all control mice to respond.
3. Treated group (which received analgesic 30 minutes. prior to clip-application) will be apathetic to pressure of clip.
4. The percentage of mice in the group that fails to respond is calculated and ED50 of the test drug is found out.

B. Material and Equipment

Hot plate (with thermostate control), Analgesic test substance.

Procedure

1. Two groups of mice are selected: one as control group and another one as treated group.
2. Both group of mice are placed on a hot plate temperature maintained at 55°C. The reaction time is between the placing the animals on the hot plate and licking of the fore or hind paws. Cut off time of 30 seconds. is followed to avoid any injury to the paws due to heat.
3. The base increase reaction time in treated group (which received analgesic substance) is calculated and ED50 value is worked out.

C. Material and Equipment

Mice restrainer cage, Radiant heat applicator. Analgesic test substance.

Procedure

1. Two groups of mice are selected : one group as control and another group as treated.
2. Mice are caged in restrainer cage with the tail protruding out. Heat transmitted by radiation is applied over the tail on a single spot with the help of radiant heat applicator. Reaction time reckons the time taken to the animal to withdraw (flick) the tail.
3. Treated group (which received analgesic 30 minutes. prior to heet application) will show higher reaction time.
4. ED50 value of the test drug can be calculated from reaction time.

Instead of radiant heat on tail, another method can be adopted. Tail up to 5 cm, is dipped in a beaker of water at 55°C. Reaction time represents the time taken to pull out the tail clearly out of water.

D. Material and Equipment

Aconitine, Analgasic test substance.

Procedure

1. Two groups of mice are selected : one group as control and another group as treated.
2. Each mouse is injected with 2 μg. of aconitine. Within 2 mins. a violent twisting or stretching syndrome, characterized by a wave of contractions of the abdominal musculature followed by extension of the hind limbs is started. This state of writhing lasts for about an hour.
3. Treated group (which received analgesic test agent 15 to 20 mins. before aconitine injection) will show protection against writhing. The percentage of protection at each dose level is calculated and ED50 value is estimated.

This writhing test is found to be selective for aspirin like analgesics. I. P. injection of phenyl quinone (0.2 ml. of 0.02% aq. soln.) or acetic acid (1 ml / 100 gms. body weight of 0.6% acetic acid) in mice will also produces same type of writhing,

EXPERIMENT 4

Motor Deficit Test in Mice

The first manifestation of depression of the CNS in the mouse is motor weakness. The present method is used in particular to test a myorelaxant, to be an antagonist of strychnins. Which is a spinal cord stimulant. This test is adaptable to a scheme including a series of methods, and especially to blind screening.

Material and Equipment

Rotating slotted cylindrical cage, Test drug.

Procedure

1. The test drug is given p. o. to groups of 10 fasted mice in geometrically increasing doses.
2. Motor weakness is detected by failure of the mice to cling to the screened side of **a** rotating, slotted cylindrical cage.
3. The ED50 dose causing motor deficit may be calculated by probit analysis and at the same time the loss of righting reflex and acute toxicity may be determined.

EXPERIMENT 5

Zwangsnagen Test in Mice

Apomorphine has unquestionable effects on mice, consequence of which leads to fearfulness, elevated motor activity and compulsive gnawing. Test may be useful for detecting substances that act on the CNS, either as depressants or stimulants or in some other way.

Material and Equipment

Apomorphine, Tin cage (30 × 45 × 20 cm., the floor is covered with corrugated paper), Test drug.

Procedure

1. Mice of either sex (18 -20 gms. body weight) is taken for this test.
2. The mice are placed in the tin cage, and gnawing is shown when the paper is removed after a given period, by the needle like holes in the corrugated paper. If a rectangular board, having the dimensions of cage and 10 rectangular windows, is placed over the paper, the number of gnawings can be estimated. The 10 windows are evenly distributed in the board according to each window covering 1% of the board's area and is divided into 10 equal smaller rectangles. Thus 100 small areas are observed and are considered as gnawed if one hole or many are present.
3. Apomorphine, 10 mg / kg body weight is given by s. c. route to one group of mice.
4. Another group of mice are given test by i. p. route and apomorphine 2 minutes, prior to test drug administration.
5. Both group of mice are placed in the cage for 1 hour. The number of smaller rectangles containing one or more holes (or greater damage) is recorded for each of the windows.
6. The mean is computed for all the windows.

EXPERIMENT 6

Nalorphine Antagonism Test in Mice

This test is designed to show morphine like properties in a drug. Nalorphine has the very attractive property of being able to do away with most of the actions of morphine. Nalorphine can displace the morphine from receptor sites and thus abolish its effects.

Material and Equipment

Nalorphine, Pirinitramide, Test drug.

Procedure

1. Mice are given a toxic dose of the test drug, followed by 0.5 - 10.0 mg/kg. nalorphine i.v. as soon as the highest point effects are observed.
2. A drug viz, pirinitramide, that caused responses such as loss of righting reflex, of the corneal reflex and of pinna reflex as well as bradypnea, had its effects antagonize in 1 minute. by an i.v. Injection of 1.25 mg *l* kg. nalorphine.

EXPERIMENT 7

Suppression of Combativeness in Mice

Some mice become fighters and temperamentally aggressive when they are isolated. Aggressive behaviour is subdued by administration of certain drugs.

Material and Equipment

Test drug.

Procedure

1. Male mice at least 4 weeks old are isolated in a cage for 3 weeks, so that no other animal can be seen. They are not disturbed except for supply of replenished food.
2. About 67% of the mice are then aggressive and will attack within 5 minutes. a non-isolated male mouse is placed in the cage. After interaction for 5 minutes. the second mouse is removed from the cage.
3. The mice of a group are given the test drug over a period of 1 – 2 weeks. 'They are tested for aggressiveness before administration and every hour for 4 hours. thereafter, on each day.
4. If no fighting occurs with the non-isolated mouse, the isolated mice are taken to have been tame and tranquillzed.

EXPERIMENT 8

Lenticular Opacity Test in Mice

Following s c. injection of narcotic analgesics in mice, at doses about 4 times the ED50 doses, determined by tail-clip method, a reversible opacity of the lens occurs. It comes to light after about ¼ hr., reaches a maximum, and then diminishes after about 3 hrs. The cloudiness appears in the lens while the cornea remains clear.

The more active the drug as an analgesic, more readily it produces an opacity. The effect of narcotic analgesic can be averted by means of simultaneous, small doses of nalorphine.

Material and Equipment

A Narcotic analgesic, Test drug.

Procedure

1. Mice of either sex, weighing 18 to 22 gms., are used.
2. Narcotic analgesic is given as aquous solutions in a constant volume of 1.0 ml/100 gms of body weight s. c. in doses from 1 to 20 mg. to mice placed in cotainers in the groups of 10.
3. The mice are examined after 15, 30, 45, 60, 75, 90, 120, 150 and 180 mins. The number of mice showing any opacity at these times is recorded.
4. The ED50 of test drug is calculated at the time of maximum activity by the method of Probit analysis.

EXPERIMENT 9

Ptosis Test in Mice

Reserpine produces ptosis in mice and this is due to central depression action. Thus central stimulants can eradicate this effect.

Material and Equipment

Reserpine, Ascorbic acid, Test drug.

Procedure

1. Male mice (18-24) gms, body weight) are selected for this ptosis test.
2. Reserpine (4mg/kg. body weight) in 5% ascorbic acid and test drug (2-3½ hrs). after reserpine) are administered by i. p. route to mice.
3. Complete ptosis is reached at about 3 hours when mice is reserpine treated.
4. The ptotic rating is made after 15 minutes. later : (a) 4 = complete ptosis ; (b) 3 = ¾ complete ; 'c) 2 = ½ complete and (d) 1 = ¼ complete, The ptosis is rated as the fraction of eyelid closure from normal aparture.
5. Two readings on each mouse are taken and averaged.

EXPERIMENT 10

Intracerebral Test in Mice

This captioned test offers a simple method to observe the efficacy of drugs introduced directly into the brain in the unanesthetized animal. Extension widely through the blood-brain is not involved. Doses are generally toned down than those are needed by other routes. Site of injection is critical : a more rostral site does not allow penetration of ventricles and a more caudal site allows too much damage to vital centre.

Material and Equipment

Hypodermic needle (3 / 8", 27 – gauge; Indian ink Test drug, saline, Surgical instruments.

Procedure

1. Groups of 10 mice (20 - 25 gms.) of either sex are used for this test.
2. Test drug is dissolved in saline and 0.01-0.05 ml, are injected.
3. The animal is grasped firmly by the loose skin in the back of the head, The skin is pulled taut. The hypodermic needle is pushed perpendicularly through the skull in the brain.
4. The site of injection is 2 mm. from the midline, on either side and on a line drawn through the anterior base of the ears.
5. For determination of the brain areas into which drug penetrates, 0.05 ml. of 1:10 dilution of Indian-ink is injected and the brains are sectioned.

   Control mice remain quiet for 1 min, and then resume normal activity.

Certain drugs cause mice

A. To assume a hunched position.

B. To Show the straub tail phenomenon.

C. To become excitable.

D. To lacrimate.

E. To salivate.

F. To become depressed.

G. To show tachypnoea.

H. To be sensitive to sound or touch.

I. To have clonic seizures.

J. To retract or draw back the ears.

K. To perkinsonian tremor.

L. To show exopthalmos.

M. To elevate the tail perpendicularly.

N. To show piloerection.

O. To show stuper.

EXPERIMENT 11

Anti-inflammatory Test by Adjuvant-Induced Arthritis is Rats

Adjuvant-induced arthritis is the only model for experiment which has often been considered to be corresponding to the human arthritic disease more closely than any other laboratory model. As such, it is always considered desirable to follow this model for screening out any anti-inflammatory agent to be of predictive value for potential use clinically. The Arthritic syndrome is induced by the intradermal injection of dead tubercle bacilli into plantar surface of right hind foot of rat,

Material and Equipment

Dead tubercle bacilli (derived from human strains), Plethysmometer. Micrometer, liquid parafin, Intradermal needle (No 20) Test drug.

Procedure

1. Two groups of pathogen free rats (200 gms. body weight) are used for adjuvant-induced arthritis test : one group serves as control & another group as treated. Right hind foots of animals are measured for thickness with the aid of micrometer across sagittal section.
2. Both groups of rats are given intradermally 0.05 ml. of fine emulsion (in liquid paraffin) of dead tubercle bacilli (5 mg */* ml) into the planter surface of right hind paw, by means of a No 20 needle.
3. Control and treated groups are given vehicle and test drug respectively for continuous 13 days, the thickness of injected foot is measured.
4. The following parameters are noted in the control and treated groups throughout the period of 14 days :
   (a) Paw Oedema by plethysmometer,
   (b) Severity of Secondary lesions (swelling of left hind paw, of the forepaws, of the ears and of the tail) is estimated as nil, mild, moderate, moderately severe and
   (c) body weight.

EXPERIMENT 12

Anti-inflammatory Test by Peritoneal Capillary Permeability in Mice

A drug's anti-inflammatory action can be screened by this test. Sustained increase that sustains in the permeability of small blood vessels to protein is a characteristic of the process of inflammation, Anti-inflammatory drugs can inhibit the exudatation of plasma proteins. probably by decreasing the permeability of small vessels. This is confirmed by observation of the inhibitory effect observed on dye leakage by causing a reduction in peritoneal capillary permeability.

Material and Equipment

Acetic acid, Saline. Pontamine sky blue, Centrifuge, Spectrocolorimeter, Test Drug, Surgical instrument.

Procedure

1. Two groups of mice are selected for this test, one for control and another as treated.
2. Control mice is given vehicle (0.1 ml.) and treated mice is given test drug by s. c, route.
3. 3 hrs. later, each mouse is given i. p. 4 ml. of 0.05 (N) acetic acid in 0.9% saline, following very quickly by 0.1 ml of 4% Pontamine sky blue, i. v.
4. 1 hr. later to the dye administration, all the animals are killed, the peritoneal cavity is opened and drained.
5. The exudate is contrifuged for 10 minutes. at 1500 g. and 0.5. ml. of the supernatant is diluted with 4.5 ml. of saline.
6. Dye concentrations are measured in a spectrocolorimeter at 625 nm. saline is used as blank.
7. The mean percentage of light absorption is then calculated for both control and drug treated groups.

EXPERIMENT 13

Anti-inflammatory Test by Carrageenin Induced Pleurisy in Rats

Migration of leucocytes is evaluated by injection of carrageenin into the pleural cavity of anaesthetized rat. Screening of anti-inflammatory drug can be carried out by this test.

Material and Equipment

Carrageenin, Hank's solution, Pasteur pipette, Haemocytometer, Microscope Test drug, Anaesthetic ether,

Procedure

1. Two groups of rats are taken : one as control and another one as treated.
2. Control and treated groups are given vechicle and test drug respectively.
3. After 30 minutes. 0.1 ml of 1% carrageenin is injected into the pleural cavity of rats which are previously anaethetized by ether.
4. After 5 hours. the animals age killed and 2 ml, of Hank's solution is injected into pleural cavity.
5. The animals are rocked to allow the mixing of the solution with the exudate.
6. Cavity is opened and the exudate is then collected with a Pasteur pipette. The total number of leucocytes present in the washing is counted with haemocytometer under microscope.

EXPERIMENT 14

Anti-inflammatory Test by Paw Oedema in Rats

oedema reckons the early phase of inflammatory condition. Carrageenin induced paw oedema is the simplest and by a large degree used model for studying the anti-inflammatory activity of new compounds. Similarly, paw oedema induced by histamine, 5-HT, bradykinin, dextran, hyaluronidase, and Prostaglan din E have been used for studying the antagonism to these mediators.

Material and Equipment

Plethysmometer, Any oedema producing agent, Test drug.

Procedure

1. Oedema producing agent (suitable conc. in saline) of 0.1 ml* volume is injected into the subplantar tissue of the rats hind foot. These animals should be considered as control,
2. Another set of rat is treated with test drug 30 minutes. Prior to the administration of oedema producing agent. This group is considered as treated.
3. Paw volume of control and treated mice are measured by plethysmometer and determination of the ED50 of the test drug is obtained by comparing the paw-volume.

EXPERIMENT 15

Anti-inflammatory Test by Cotton Pellet Granuloma in Rats

Germ free cotton is implanted along the flanks or axillae of rats. Granuloma is measured by weighment of the implanted cotton pellet after removal. Screening of anti-infammatory drug can be conducted by the test.

Material and Equipment

Cotton pellets, Dryer, Test drug, Anaesthetic ether, Surgical instruments.

Procedure

1. Two groups of rats are selected for this granuloma test; one for control and another for treatment. Both group of rats are anaesthetized by ether.
2. Sterile cotton balls (weighing 10 mg. each) are implanted s.c. allong ths flanks or axillae of both group of rats,
3. Control rats are given vehicle (0.2 ml.) and treated rats are given test drus by i.p. route for 7 days from the day of cotton pellet implantation.
4. Granuloma is measured by weighing the implanted cotton pellets after their removal, on the 8th day.
5. The pellets are freed from extraneous tissues and dried at 60°C in a forced air dryer to constant weight.

EXPERIMENT 16

Anti-inflammatory Test by Inflammatory Exudation in Mice

Perintoneal inflammation can be produced in mice by administration of acetic acid in peritoneal cavity. Measuring of the degree of exudation of inflammation can be evoluated. Screening of anti-inflammatory drug can be done by this method of test.

Material and Equipment

Acetic acid, Di-NaEDTA, Physiological saline Centrifuge, spectrocolorimeter, Biuret reagent. Test drug, Surgical instruments.

Procedure

1. Selection is made of two groups of mice: one for control and another for treatment.
2. Control mice are given vehicle (0.1 ml.) and treated mice are given teat drug by i. p. route.
3. After 30 minutes, 0.25 ml. of 1.2% acetic acid is given to each mouse by i, p. route.
4. After 3 hours., inner parts of this animal body is exposed by abdominal cutting. And abdomen is washed with physiological saline containing 0.1 ml, disodium EDTA. The volume of each washing is made upto 6 ml, with physiological saline and then centrifuge at 1500 r. p. m.
5. The total amount of protein in the supernatant fluid is estimated with Biuret reagent in a spectrocolorimeter.

EXPERIMENT 17

Antipyretic Test in Rats

This test is carried out for screening of antipyretic agent.

Material and Method

Dry Yeast, Gastric tube, Electronic thermometer, Test substance.

Procedure

1. Rats are made hyperthermic by s. c. injection (1 ml/100gms. body weight) of a 12% suspension of dry yeast.
2. 10 hrs later the animals are given the test substance by gastric tube. The mean temperature for group is ascertained definitely by means of electronic thermometer at 90, 180 and 270 minutes. after the dose of test substance.
3. The difference between the mean temperature of the control group and that of other group is calculated.

EXPERIMENT 18

Hyaluronidase Inhibition in Mice

This test is designed to gauge inhibition of hyaluronidase activity, which often stands parallel to anti-inflammatory activity. Hgaluronidase also accilerates the absorption of drug administered by s c. route. This method is described quantitative although it may easily be adapted to a qualitative screening procedure.

Material and Equipment

Hyaluronidase, Urethan, Sodium hydroxide, Test drug.

Procedure

1. Female mice (20 - 22 gms. body weight) are used in groups of five.
2. Room temperature is kept at 21°C - 22°C. Urethan as 10% aqueous solution is given by s. c. in a dose of 1.2 mg/gm. of body weight.
3. The time from the injection to the moment when the animal offers no resistance to being placed on its side, is noted and recorded as the absorption time of urethane.
4. A dose of 0.01 ml/gm of body weight of a hyaluronidase solution containing 380 TRU ml (turbitity reducing units) is injected i. v. into tail veins of another group.
5. 2 minutes. later the animals are given urethane by s. c., as described above. The time for absorption is diminished for this group.
6. To test inhibitory activity, the test drug is dissolved in dilute sodium hydroxide at pH 7, 40 minutes before the injection of hyaluronidase, the test drug is given by s. c. or p. o. route.
7. The minimum dose necessary to inhibit completely the reduction of the absorption time caused by hyaluronidase is expressed as MID 100 (minimul inhibitory dose).
8. Controls are groups of mice being given saline and urethane or saline, hyaluronidase and urethan.

EXPERIMENT 19

Effect of Vagal Stimulation and of Histamine on Gastric Secretion of Rats

Material and Equipment

Histamine solution (100 mg / cc) ; Standard Sodium hydroxide, approx 0.0l(N), Anaesthetic Ether, Phenolphthalein 1% in 50 % alcohol.

Procedure

Two rats are used, Rat I for vagal stimulation and Rat II for histamine injection.

1. The rats are anaesthetized
2. In Rat I, one of the vagi in the neck is exposed.
3. The pyloric end of the stomachs of Rats I and I1 are cannulated and by means of a syringe filled with saline warmed to body temperature, the gastric content is throughly washed out.
4. The cannulae is clamped off and the incisions are closed with wound clips.
5. The rats are kept warm and the wounds are coveted with warm saline packs. Then stomachs are washed out thoroughly and the washing are titrated with standard NaOH to determine the normal secretion of hydrochloric acid.
6. The cannulae is clamped off the wounds are closed.
7. In Rat I, the vagus is tied off and cut.
8. During the ensuing 30 minutes the distal end is stimulated for 5 secs, and 20 seconds. intervals.
9. At the end of that time the stomach is again washed out and the washings are titrated.
10. Rat I1 injected s.c. with 100 mg / kg. of histamine.
11. After 30 mins, the stomach is washed out and the washings are titrated.

EXPERIMENT 20

The Secretion and Digestive Action of Pancreatic Juice of Rats

In the first part of this experiment, the action of secretion in stimulating pancreatic juice secretion is demonstrated, In the second part, the digestive action of trypsin on protein is studied.

Material and Equipment

Intestinal cannula, Bile duct cannula.

(Made by attaching a short length of 22-gauge hypodermic needle, with blunt, rounded end, to an 8 cm. piece of 24-gauge Transflex tubing. The tubing should be marked at 5 mm. intervals.)

Mett's tubes.

(Capillary tubes such as used for blood coagulation.)

Incubator (at 37° C-40° C.)

50 cc. of 5 percent hydrochloric acid.

50 cc. of 10 % sodium hydroxide.

White of egg.

Pilocarpine solution, 0.75 mg/cc,

Buffer solution, pH 8.4.

(Dissolve 12.405 gm. of boric acid and 14.912 gm. of potassium chloride in 1 liter of water. To 50 cc, of this solution add 8.5cc of 0.2 N sodium hydroxide.)

Procedure Part-I

1. In the rat, many of the pancreatic ducts empty into the bile duct. This may be demonstrated by cannulating the bile duct as described below and injecting a solution of methylene blue, which, by filling the pancreatic ducts, makes them readily visible.
2. A rat is anaesthetized with Nembutal, and one jugular vein cannulated. A transverse incision is made, beginning at the border of the lower ribs on the right side and extending to the mid line. The bile duct is located and its upper end is tied off just below its

bifurcation. The duct is traced toward the intestine. The lower end is seen lying along the surface of the intestine. Now a cut is made in the intestinal wall just below the point where the bile duct disappears. Cannulation is performed by inserting the tip of the cannula into the bile duct through the cut in the intestinal wall. A thread is passed around the bile duct by means of a curved needle, and the cannula tied in place. (It is necessary that the cannulation be made very low in order to prevent tying off one of the largest of the entering pancreatic ducts,)

3. The pancreatic juice has risen in the cannuls, and the rate of flow is determined by timing its rise past 2 or 3 of the marked divisions of the cannula. This represents the normal secretion rate.
4. Another rat is sacrificed and the entire small intestine is excised. The intestine is filled with 5 % hydrochloric acid and allowed to stand for 1 hour. The intestinal content is removed, boiled for several minutes and neutralized with 10 % sodium hydroxide and filtered.
5. The secretin solution is warmed to body temperature, and 1 cc. is slowly injected into the jugular vein.

Procedure Part - II

1. Another rat is anaesthetized, and a transverse incision made as described above. A loop of the small intestine is now cannulated, one cannula being inserted just below the pyloric sphincter and the other about 2 cm. below the entrance of the bile duct.
2. The upper end of bile duct is tied off just below its bifurcation, to prevent the entrance of bile.
3. The intestinal loop between the cannula is washed out with warm saline, which is discarded.
4. The intestinal caunula are now clamped off for 30 minutes, following which the intestinal loop is washed out with exactly 5 cc. of warm saline. This represents the control enzyme solution.
5. Now 1 cc/kg of the pilocarpine solution is directly introduced into the abdominal cavity. After 30 minutes, the intestinal loop is washed out again with 5 cc. of warm saline. This represents the experimental solution.

6. The white of an egg is strained through fine cheesecloth and it is drawn up into the capillary tubes. The tubes ate held horizontally and these are dropped into water at 85°C. The water cooled. The end of the tubes are sealed with paraffin. in which condition they will keep indefinitely:
7. To the control and experimental enzyme solutions, now equal volumes of the buffer solution are added. The capillary tubing containing the coagulated egg white are cut into 2 cm. sections and these are placed in small test tubes which have been filled with the enzyme soluions, These are placed in the incubator (37° C– 40° C,) for 48 hrs.

EXPERIMENT 21

Gastric Motility Test by Charcoal Meal in Mice

The Charcoal meal is given to mice. And the mice are sacrificed to measure the passage of charcoal meal in intestine. Any drug which influences the motility of the intestine can be measured by this model.

Material and Equipment

Animal Charcoal, Tragacanth, Oral needle, Test drug, Surgical instruments.

Procedure

1. Adult mice. (20 gms.-25 gms.) are given Charcoal meal (animal Charcoal 12 gms., tragacanth 2 gms, and water 130 ml.) by oral needle.
2. After 15 minutes. the mice are killed.
3. The abdomen is opened.
4. The small intestine from pylorus to ileocaecal juncton is dissected out.
5. The distance which the charcoal meal travels can be measured and expressed as a percentage of the total length of small intestine.
6. Passage of charcoal in both normal and treated mice is recorded and ED50 of the test drug is calculated.

EXPERIMENT 22

Gastric Ulceration by Pylorus Ligation in Rats

Rats are used for evaluation of various agents for production of gastric ulcer.

Material and Equipment

Anaesthetic ether, Bent needle, Formalin Soln. Light microscope, Surgical instruments, 'Test drug.

Procedure

1. Rat weighing 140-165 gms. are housed in individual cages and fasted for 48 hours, before pyloric ligation. Water is supplied ad libitum.
2. Care should be taken to avoid coprophagy.
3. Rats are anaesthetised by ether and abdomen is opened by small middle incision below the xiphoid process pyloric portion of the stomach is slightly lifted out and ligated avoiding traction to the pylorus or damage to its blood supply.
4. The stomach is replaced carefully and the abdominal wall closed by interrupted sutures.
5. Test drug is administered s.c. once daily for 2 days prior to and immediately after pyloric ligation.
6. The rats are deprived of both food and water during the postoperative period and are sacrificed at the end of 19 hrs. following operation.
7. The stomach is dissected out and the contents from the stomach are draind into a tube and this is subjected to analysis of pH and for free and total acidity.
8. The stomach is then cut open along the greater curvature and the inner and outer layer is fixed in formalin solution.
9. Inner surface is examined microscopically to detect any ulceration. And the degree of ulceration is measured by following the method of scoring

Necrohaemorrhagic spots greater than 2 mm. diameter are taken as ulcers. These are graded as follows :

0.5 = minute, sporadic punctuate lesions;

1 = Several small lesions;

2 = One lesion of extension or multiple moderate sized lesions;

3 = several large lesions.

EXPERIMENT 23

Test of Antiulcer Agents by Cold Restraint Ulcer (CRU) in Rats

Gastric ulceration in rat can be induced by keeping the animal in cold (4°C) and in immobilized condition. The efficacy of drugs to protect this ulceration can be observed in this model.

Material and Equipment

Anaesthetic ether. wire mesh, 1% Formalin, Light microscope, Surgical instruments, Test drug.

Procedure

1. Male rats weighing 110- 160 gms. are fasted for 36 -40 hours. (only water allowed *ad libttum.)*
2. Rats are lightly anaesthetised by ether and immobilised by folding and securing wire mesh around animals' body.
3. After recovery from anaesthesia they are placed supine at 4°C for 3 hrs.
4. Following 3 hrs. cold plus restraint stress (CRS\, the rats are sacrificed and stomachs are removed.
5. The stomachs are cut along greater curvature and inner and outer layer is fixed by instillation of 1% formalin solution.
6. Inner layer of the stomachs is examined by a light microscope.
7. Severity of the growth of ulcer an arbitrary scoring system is used to determine "Ulcer index".
8. Scoring system of ulcer determination is as follows :
    1. Denuded epithelial = 10,
    2. Petechial and frank haemorrohages = 20,
    3. One or two ulcers- 30,
    4. Multiple ulcer = 40,
    5. Perforated ulcers=50.

EXPERIMENT 24

Liver Function' Tests of Rats

One test for liver function is the rate of removal of the dye, bromsulphalein, from the blood. . In this experiment the retardation of removal is demonstrated with liver function is impaired.

Material and Equipment

Instruments for cannulation Trachea carotid, and jugular cannula for bile duct, Bromsulphalein (BSP) solutions (2mg/c,c; and 0.02 mg/c.c).

0.l(N) NaOH, Stop watch, Colorimeter, Centrifuge,

Procedure

1. The treachea, left carotid artery, and right jugular vein are cannulated and heparinized.
2. The bile duct is also cannulated.
3. 0.5 c.c, of blood is collected from the carotid artery and transfered to a 15c.c.centrifuge tube.
4. BSP is injected via the jugular vein (5 mg./kg.) ; the stop watch is started A small dish containing a few c c. of 0.1 (N) NaOH is placed under the end of the bile cannula. The BSP is removed from the blood stream by the liver and excreted in the bile. When the bile containing the BSP comes in contact with the alkali it turns to 'purple 'color'; the first dye' appears in 3 -4 mins.
5. Two mins. after the injection of BSP another 0.5 C.C. sample of blood is collected and transfered to the second centrifuge tube.
6. After about 30 mins., during which time most of the dye has been removed from the blood, two lobes of the liver are clamped off with hemostats so as to reduce the effectiveness of the liver.
7. The injection of BSP is repeated as in part 4,
8. A 0.5 c.c. sample of blood is collected 2 minutes after the BSP injection, 2nd is transfered to a third centrifuge tube.
9. The three blood samples are centrifuged, 0.2 c.c. of plasma is measured from each, and is transfered to test tubes.

10. To the first test tube 2.0 c.c. of H_2O, 0.5 c.c. of the BSP solution containing 0.02 mg/c.c. and 3.0 c.c. of 0.1 (N) NaOH are added. To tubes 2 and 3, 2 5 c.c. of H_2O and 3 c c. of 0 1 (N) NaOH are added.
11. The resulting solutions are compared in a calorimeter.
12. The % retention of the dye in an animal with normal liver function is calculated and when a portion of the liver was clamped off the plasma volume is assumed to be 3% of the body weight.

EXPERIMENT 25

Liver Cancer Model in Rats

Liver carcinoma can be produced in rat by administering chemical carcinogen, diethyl nitrosoamine along with 2-amino acetyl fluorine, The later chemical is used here as a malignancy promoter.

Material and Equipment

Oral needle, Diethyl Nitrosoamine (DENA), 2 - Amino Acetyl fluorine (2 - AAF), Surgical instruments.

Procedure

1. Two groups of rats (150-175 gms. body weight) are selected for this model, one for control and another for treated. Each group contains 5 rats.
2. Partial hepatoctomy (3/4th) is done in both groups of rats.
3. After 18 hours of hepatoctomy, DENA is given p .o. by oral needle to treated group at the single dose level of 35 mg/kg. body weight. Control group is given only vehicle.
4. The treated group is given drinking water added with 0.02%, 2-AAF for 12 weeks from the 6th week after DENA treatment, This 2 - AAF is acted as malignancy promoter.
5. After 4 - 5 months of above treatments rats are dissected out for confirmation of liver malignancy. Malignant liver will develop. The number of foci will vary from 6 - 12 on the 5th month.

Afterwards the foci will further increase in number. Further more, all the tissues growing across the hepatoctomized liver will become malignant. The pale grey color of the liver (completely malignant) will appear at about 30 weeks and onwards.

Another potent carcinogenic chemical know as diethyl amino benzene (DEAB) is used to produce liver cancer in rat. Within 3 – 4 months, this chemical produces liver carcinoma in rat. And if this chemical is used, no hepatoctomy is necessary.

EXPERIMENT 26

Kidney Function Tests of Rats

It has been shown that PSP (phenol red) is removed from the circulation almost entirely by the kidney and damage to the kidney will decrease the rate at which the dye is excreted. This experiment is designed to demonstrate the use of PSP in the determination of kidney function.

Material and Equipment

Instruments for cannulation Trachea, Carotid, and Jugular cannula, Phenolsulfonephthalein (PSP) solutions.

0.1(N)NaOH,

Stop watch,

Colorimeter,

Centrifuge,

Procedure

1. The trachea, left carotid artery, and right jugular vein are cannulated and are heparinized.
2. Renal artery and renal vein are dissected out to one kidney and one loop of thread is placed around the two vessels. It is not tied.
3. 0.5 c.c. of blood from the carotid artery is removed and transfered to a centrifuge tube, This sample is used to make the standard for colorimetric analysis.
4. Injection of 5 mg/kg. of PSP via the jugular vein is done and the stop watch is stprted.
5. Exactly 2 minutes after the injection of the PSP, collection of 0.5 c.c. of blood is done and it is transfered to a second centrifuge tube.
6. After about 30 minutes, the blood flow is prevented to one kidney by tightening the loop of thread previously placed around thermal vessels.
7. The injection of 5 mg./kg. of PSP is repeated and exactly 2 minutes, after the injection, another 0.5 c.c, sample of blood is transfered to a third centrifuge tube.
8. The three blood samples are centrifuged, 0.2 c.c, of plasma from each is measured and transfered to numbered test tubes.

9. To the first tube standard 1.5 c.c. of water, 1.0 c.c, the PSP solution containing 0.006 mg/c.c. and 3 c.c. of 0.1 (N) NaOH are added. To tubes 2 and 3, 2.5 c. c. of water and 3 c. c. of 0.1 (N) NaOH are added respectively.
10. The resulting solutions are compared in a calorimeter
11. The percentage retention of the dye is calculated when there is normal kidney function and when the circulation to one kidney has been impaired. Assume the plasma volume to be 3 percent of the body weight.

EXPERIMENT 27

Saline Diuresis in Rats

In this experiment the effect of intravenous injections of saline and of a 10% glucose solution upon the rate of urinary excretion is observed.

Material and Equipment

Small-bore glass cannula for urethral cannulation (with one end bent at right angles)

Procedure

The rat used in this experiment should have been placed on a "wet" diet (bread and milk, lettuce, carrots) for several days before this experiment.

1. A jugular vein is cannulated and the wound is closed temporarily with clips.
2. A mid-line incision is made through the lower third of the abdomen and the pelvic viscera is exposed. The urinary bladder lies just anterior to the symphysis pubis.
3. It is not necessary to cut the symphysis ; by carefully clearing away the overlying muscle and connective tissue a sufficient length of the urethra is exposed.

   Cannulation is done, being sure that the tip of the cannula lies freely within the bladder and with the bent end extending downward between the rat's hind legs.
4. The wound is closed with clips, being careful not to disturb the position of the cannula. The wound is kept warm and moist without exterting pressure on it.
5. The urinary flow during a 15 minutes. period is observed and there will not be more than a drop or two and perhaps not any.
6. 5 c.c, of saline solution, warmed to body temperature is slowly injected into the jugular vein. The drops of urine secreted over 5 minutes intervals are counted during the next 20 minutes. If the first 5c.c. of the saline are not effective, the injection is repeated.
7. After the diuresis has ceased and the flow returned to normal, 1 c.c, of a 10% glucose solution is injected. An even more marked diuresis follows (The rat is highly resistant to the diuretic action of caffeine, and relatively resistant to urea).

EXPERIMENT 28

Production of Renal Hypertension of Rats

This experiment introduces a method for the experimental production of hypertension by compression of the kidney. This compression results in a reduction of blood flow, in consequence of which the kidney secretes a vasopressor agent known as "renin."

The so-called "tail method" of determining blood pressure is employed.

Material and Equipment

Blood pressure apparatus, Sterile gauze, Cellulose acerate.

Procedure

Young (100 gms-125 gms.) rats are used. Since the blood pressure determination takes only a few minutes, tame rats, held lightly covered with a towel, usually remain quiet during the test ; or they map be lightly anaesthetized with Nembutal (25mg/kg). Several determinations are made on each rat, and the results averaged. They are then rendered hypertensive, as described below, and the blood pressure determinations repeated some 30 days later.

The blood pressure is determined as follows :

1. The cuff around the rat's tail 1 cm. distal is placed to the root.
2. The cap of the metal gland is removed and it is packed with soft soap. The cap is replaced with the thread lightly engaged. The central core of soap is removed, i. e., that lying between the two drilled holes. The plethysmograph is attached to the gland by means of a short rubber tube, one end of which fits over the plethysmograph tube and the other inserts snugly into the large drilled hole of the gland.
3. The rat's tail is inserted into the plethysmograph through the small drilled hole to within 2 cm, of the cuff. The cap of the gland is screwed down until the tail is engaged by the Soap
4. The circulation is arrested by rapid inflation of the cuff to a pressure above the systolic level.
5. The plethysmograph is filled with water at about 40°C and the level is adjusted in the capillary to a convenient point.

6. The pressure is allowed to fall slowly by means of the release valve of the bulb, watching the level of fluid in the capillary tube meanwhile. When the systolic pressure is passed, an abrupt rise in the capillary tube will occur. The pressure may then be read from the manometer.

The method for producing renel hypertension is described below. However, this operation must be performed under sterile conditions, since the animals are to be kept alive for some time.

1. The rat is anaesthetized with Nembutal.
2. The animal is placed in a prone position and a dorsal midline incision is made extending from about TI0 to 13.
3. The skin is deflected to the sides & dissection is made through The thin muscle walls just anterior to the upper poles of the kidneys. The kidneys are lifted from their beds, and the surrounding fat are cleared away. The pad of fat at the upper pole, enclosing the adrenal gland, is freed very carefully.
4. The kidneys are encircled with sterile gauze, applying the first layer parallel to the long axis of the kidney. Furthet layers are applied circularly, care being taken not to close blood vessels
5. The gauze is coated with several layers of thin cellulose acetate, permitting each coat to dry before applying the next. Drying is rapid only a minute or two being required for each coat.
6. The kidneys are replaced, the muscle wound is closed with sutures and the skin incision with wound clips.

EXPERIMENT 29

The Rate of Glucose Absorption in Rats

In this experiment the rate of absorption of glucose, expressed in terms of the Cori and Cori coefficient, namely, the number of milligrams per 100 gms of rat per hour, is determined.

Material and Equipment

Syringe and needle for oral administration. Reagents for Schaffer-Somogyi method for sugar determination.

1. 5 gms, of glucose per kilogram body weight, in a 50% solution is administered orally to a rat which has been starved for 24 hrs.
2. After 2 hours, the rat is killed the esophagus is tied off at the cardiac sphincter and the small intestine at the iliocolic sphincter, and the stomach and small intestine are removed, The blood is washed from the outside. The tract is slit open and the content is washed out thoroughly with water.
3. It is filtered, diluted to 400 c.c., and *5* c.c. aliquots is measured into large Pyrex test tubes 5 C.C. of water is measured into a test tube and treated in the same manner as the unknowns.
4. 5 c.c. of the copper reagent is added to each tube, washing down the sides : the samples are mixed and covered with one hole rubber stoppers to avoid oxidation.
5. It is placed in a boiling water bath for 15 minutes with as little agitation as possible.
6. It cooled in running water and 2 cc. of the KI-K2C204 solution and 5 cc. of (N) sulfuric acid are added. It is covered with a small beaker and agitated.
7. After a few minutes the beakers are washed into the test tubes and titrated with 0.005 (N) sodium thiosulfate solution, made by diluting the 0.1 (N) 2-3 drops of the starch solution are added when the brown iodine color became yellow and the titration is continued until the starch blue is gone and the delicate copper green is visible.

EXPERIMENT 30

Alloxan Diabetes in Rats

Since the pancreas in the rat is diffuse structure, the production of diabetes by pancreatectomy is difficult. In this experiment, diabetes is produced by the injection of alloxan, a drug which has a specific destructive action on the islets of Langerhans.

Material and Equipment

Alloxan solution containing 100 mg / c.c,

Reagents for the Folin Malmros sugar determination method.

Procedure

1. The rate used are starved for 48 hrs.
2. These are anaesthetized lightly with Nembutal.
3. A sample of tail blood is obtained for normal blood sugar determination.
4. Alloxen is injected i.p. in a dose of 300 mg / kg. (containing100 mg / c. c.)
5. After 24 hours another sample of tail blood is obtained. It is found that a marked degree of hyperglycemia bas been produced. If desired, the test may be repeated the following day ; the blood sugar will be found to be even higher.

EXPERIMENT 31

Effect of Insulin on Sugar of Rats

Material and Equipment

Insulin solution containing 2 units per cubic centimeter.

The regular, not modified insulin should be used, Reagents for Folin-Malmros sugar-determination method

Procedure

1. The animals used have been starved for 48 hours.
2. They are anaesthetized lightly with Nembutal.
3. A sample of tail blobs has been taken for the normal sugar determination.
4. 2 Units of insulin/kg. is injected, i. p.
5. After 30 minutes, samples of tail blood is taken, The rats map or may not be in convulsions, but have at hand 5% glucose solution to relieve the hypoglycemic shock. After the samples have been taken, glucose is injected i. p.
6. The amount of glucose in the samples is determined by means of the Folin-Malmros method.

EXPERIMENT 32

Preparation of Septal Lesions in Rats

It is quite likely that rats having bilateral lesions of septal area may be of use in screening antidepressant agents. Septal rat shows behavioural abnormalities like exaggerated reactions to a puff of air, to the approach of a glove and to handling Since a calming action caused by a test compound can be exposition of ataxia, evaluation of compounds are made both by their effects on the rage-like behaviour and on the ability of normal rats to remain on a rotating wooden rod, where they have been trained to walk previously. The ED50's for calming and for inability to remain on the rod are compared.

Material and Equipment

Anaesthetic ether, Bent sewing needle, 90° bent needle.

Procedure

1. Normal adult rats (150-250 gms.) are taken.
2. Anaesthetic ether is applied for anaesthetising rats, the periosteum of the cranium is resected. About 0.5 mm. behind the frontal pole of cerebral hemisphere, a small hole is drilled on the mid-line, through cranium.
3. A needle, with its tip bent to make an angle of 90° with the shaft, and subsequently sharpened is pushed into the hole to a measured depth, which is approximately to the central region of brain.
4. Rotation of needle for a few times is needed to produce a bilateral lesion before it being withdrawn. The periosteum is sewed over the hole, and then the skin sewed together. No bandage is used.
5. Within 2 hours after the operation the animals show great changes in behaviour. The limbs are rigidly extended ; the eyes follow moving objects intensely ; auditory stimuli are very startling, and attempts to handle the animal cause vigorous attack or flight.

EXPERIMENT 33

Production of Anaphylactic Shock in Rats

Although the rat is markedly resistant to sensitization, anaphylactic shock may almost invariably be produced by the technique described in this experiment.

Material and Equipment

Normal horse serum, Blood pressure setup.

Procedure

1. To sensitize, the rats are injected i. p. with 2 c.c. of horse serum per rat per injection, at 3 day intervals. for 3 injections. 15 days following the last injection the test for anaphylactic shock is carried out.
2. Cannulation of carotid artery and the opposite jugular vein is done.
3. Carotid cannula is attached to the tambour, and, while a normal record is being taken. 0.25 C.C. of horse serum (warmed to body temperature) is injected into the jugular vein. An extreme fall in blood pressure will occur either immediately or within a few minutes; the heart may stop and respiration cease. The animal can sometimes be revived by administering artificial respiation.
4. To prove that sensitization was responsible, a control experiment is carried out using an unsensitized rat. It is found that the injection of 0.25 c.c. of horse serum produces no such effect.

EXPERIMENT 34

Oxytocin Cramping in Rats

Oxytocin, the hormone of the posterior pituitary gland that causes uterine contractions, leads to "Cramping" in rats. The cramping response consists of abdominal contractions stretching of the trunk and hind limbs and torsion of the body at the hips with inward rotation of one hind foot. The response may be eliminated by prior administration of morphine and related substances, for which the ED50 is much less than that found with a procedure using radiant heat. The test is thus deemed more sensitive.

Material and Equipment

Diethylstilboestrol, Oxytocin, Test drug.

Procedure

1. Female rats (120 - 140 gms. body weight) are treated with estrogen by implanting a I5 mg pellet of diethylstilboestrol s. c. in the thigh of the animal. After 10 weeks the animals are ready for this analgesic test,
2. The test drug is administered s. c. 15 minutes, before an i. p. dose of 2 units of Oxytocin (an ED50 dose),
3. Groups of 10 rats are used. The % decrease in the incidence of cramping, is determined, and the ED50 value is estimated.

EXPERIMENT 35

A Test of Suppression of a Conditioned Response in Rats

To obtain this method, the stainless steel gridfloor in a wooden box becomes the source of electrical shocks to rats, which can escape the noxious stimulus by climbing a centrally located wooden pole. The stimulus is approximately 0.1 mA of 60 cycle alternating current at 40 volts. The conditioning stimulus is a buzzer attached to the chamber.

Material and Equipment

Condition response box, Test drug.

Procedure

1. Female rats, (175 - 295 gms) are trained by a shock of duration by 30 seconds to climb the pole. They are later conditioned to do likewise at the sound of bazzer, of 12 secs, duration.
2. Satisfactorily trained and conditioned rats, in group of 10, are given i, p. doses of the test drug.
3. At hourly interval thereafter, for 5 hours the response of each animal to the buzzer is ascertainable by 3 successive trials.
4. The inhibition of the conditioned response stands as a measure of the tranquillization.
5. A dose response curve prepared in the usual way allows the calculation of ED50.

EXPERIMENT 36

Palpebral Test in Rats

The object of this test is to weigh the tendency of the animal to withdraw or to go into the resting state, such as preceding sleep. Thus depression of CNS and relaxation are measured. The test is subjective but may serve as a quick screening method. Morphine, amphetamine create exophthalmia in rats, while CNS depressants produce some palpebral closure.

Material and Equipment

Test Drug.

Procedure

1. Eight pairs of male adult rats are selected.
2. One member of each pair is given the drug s. c. ; the other member, the vehicle.
3. After 1 hour., the animals, housed alone in cages, are observed by 2 trained observers.
4. The observers without physical touch of rats select the rat of a pair having the greater tendency of shutting eyes, i, e. the rat having smaller palpebral aperture.
5. The system of scoring is given below :

To select that animal of each pair which shows the less general motor activity ; To score 1 for failure to observe a significant difference in activity, so that a clear selection can be made. To score 2 for a clear difference made unhesitatingly ; To score 3 if the difference is due to drug action.

EXPERIMENT 37

Runway Test for Thirsty Rats

Thirsty rats are trained in this test to run a 2 m. runway to water. This test along with rotating rod test may provide some means of distinguishing an antidepressant property of test drug from a property of tranquilising effect.

Material and Equipment

Runway box (a starting box 12 × 30 cm ; and alley (narrow passage) 12 × 120 cm. ; a reward box 12 × 30 cm.) ; Test drug.

Procedure

1. 10 rats are studied at each dose level. The animals are trained until the total time from being put into box till they reach the water, which is approximately 2-3 seconds. The period of training stretches over 6 - 10 days.
2. Each animal is given two control trails preceding the appropriate i. p. injection.
3. At each 30 mins. interval following the injection, the animals are given one test trial. The latency (the time from being put into the starting box to the exit from first door) is found to be the most sensitive to drug effect. The drug effect on latency is expressed as the percent of animal which have a latency of 10 secs. Or longer.
4. The runway ED50 is calculated for each compound by Probit analysis.

EXPERIMENT 38

Test for Dermal Absorption in Rats

The absorption through the skin may be influenced by various compounds. This test may be of use in showing the effect of a compound on the absorption rate.

Material and Equipment

Rat Cage, glass cylinder, wax and paraffin, 0.5%, KCN solution, Compound 48/80, Soap.

Procedure

1. Male rats (220 gms. body weight) are used in this test.
2. They are placed on round shaped rat-cage from which the tails hang free outside the cage.
3. The tail is washed with soap. dried, and placed in a glass cylinder containing 0.5% KCN at pH 8.5.
4. The root of the tail is covered with a mixture of wax and paraffin (1:1 ratio) so that the body does not contact the solution. The cylinder is maintained at 30°C.
5. Under the indicated circumstances the control rats die after 4.42 hrs, as a result of subcutaneous absorption of KCN.
6. Rats which are given compound 48/80, a histamine releasing agent, for 6 days in increasing i p. doses (100, 150, 200, 250, 300,350 mg/100 gms. body weight) die after 8 hours
7. Thus histamine, when released so that it leaves the skin, lessens the absorption through the skin. Other substance may diminish absorption or accelerate it which can be estimated from survival time of rats.

EXPERIMENT 39

Lacrimation Test in Rats

This test is designed to exhibit parasympathetic blockade and its reversal, as demonstrated by lacrimation.

Material and Equipment

Carbamylcholine, A piece of Cotton, Test drug.

Procedure

1. Rat (150 - 225 gms. body weight) are used in this test.
2. The animals are kept at 36°C for 10 minutes. before use with a view to causing vasodilatation.
3. The test drug is thereafter injected into the tail vein, the volume of solution being 1 ml /kg. body weight, and duration of the injection being 20 seconds.
4. A dose of 0.5 mg/kg. carbamylcholine is given i. p. after 15,45,75 and 105 minutes. or until a positive response is obtained.
5. The appearance of a coloured spot on a piece of cotton pressed over the eye, within 3 minutes. after injection of carbamylcholine, is taken as a positive response. Failure to obtain a coloured spot at proper time interval is considered parasympatholytic activity.
6. The ED50 of test drug, the dose necessary to prevent the appearance of a coloured spot in half of the animals after 105 minutes is estimated.

EXPERIMENT 40

The Effects of Adrenalectomy and the Action of Cortin in Rats

The group of experiments on the endocrine system includes a number of 'chronic' experiments, i, e., operations following which the animals are to be kept alive for an indefinite period. Such operations must be performed under sterile conditions, to avoid wound infection.

Experiment on the Adrenal Cortex

In this experiment the fact that the adrenal cortex is necessary to maintain life demonstrated by removing the adrenal glands from a group of rats ; half the group is left untreated and dies within a week, the other half receives a potent preparation of cortical hormone and is found to remain in good condition as long as the injections are continued.

Material and Equipment

Sterile pack, Surgical instruments, Cortin preparation.

Procedure

1. Preparation has been made for the operation as described above. Male rats weighing 45-55 gms. should be used.
2. With the rat on the prone position a dorsal mid-line incision about 2 cm. long is made, extending from about the tenth thoracic to the third lumbar vertebra. Both adrenals are removed from this central skin incision.
3. The skin retracted laterally to the right and, with a pair of fine pointed forceps, a small hole is forced through the thin muscle wall just anterior to the upper pole of the kidney. The forceps are pulled open to enlarge the hole. The adrenal is imbedded in fat and connective tissue, which is loosely attached to the upper pole of the kidney.
4. Grasping the fat surrounding the adrenal with one forceps, it is dissected loose from the kidney with the points of another. The gland itself is not touched, as it is friable and easily crushed. In rats of this size the blood vessels supplying the adrenal are small and so it is not needed to be ligated. The mass of fat is lifted out of the wound and it is examined to be sure it contains the adrenal.

5. The muscle wound is closed with one or two stiches, using fine silk thread and a curved needle.
6. The operation is repeated on the left size and the skin incision is closed with wound clips.
7. The operated animals are divided into two groups ; the untreatedgroup is weighed daily and watched for symptoms of cortical deficiency. A progressive loss in body weight and, within a few days, anorexia, weakness, and a reduction in body temperature are noted, ending in death, usually between the fifth and eighth days.
8. The members of the treated group are injected with 0.25 mg. of Cortin daily for a 10 day period, beginning the day after the operation. The injection is made s. c. and the rats are weighed at the time of injection. This dose is adequate to maintain normal growth and health.
9. At the end of that period injections are discontinued; the rats deteriorated, and death followed. An occasional rat survived indefinitely, owing either to incomplete operative removal or to the existence of accessory cortical tissue.

EXPERIMENT 41

Mode of Action of Gonadotropic Hormones in Rats

In this experiment the fact is demonstrated that the action of gonadotropic hormones in stimulating accessory sex organs is indirect, i. e., by way of the gonads. Chorionic hormone, either from pregnancy urine or from pregnant mare serum is used rather than anterior lobe gonadotropin, as the latter is relatively ineffective in stimulating seminal vesicle growth.

Material and Equipment

Sterile pack and surgical instruments, Gonadotropic .hormone preparation.

Procedure

Four groups of rats are studied.

Group 1. Immature females (30 days old) are injected daily for 3 days with a total dose of 20 I. U. of gonadotropic hormone and killed at the end of 100 hrs. following the first injection. The vagina is found to have opened, and a positive estrus smear, is obtained. Enlargement and distention of the uterus are also noted.

Group 2. This group is ovariectomized, as previously described, at the age of 21 days, and a week or 10 days later is given the same course of injections as Group 1 Examination at the end of 100 hours. showed none of the maturation effects seen in Group 1, proving that the gonadotropic hormone produced its effect by way of ovaries.

Group 3. These group consists of young males, 30 days old. They are injected in the same way as the previous groups and killed at the end of 100 hours. The seminal vesicles dissected out and weighed.

Group 4. This animals are castrated, when about 21 days old, given a week or so for recovery, and then injected as above. Seminal vesicles are dissected out and weighed. The increased weight of the seminal vesicles of Group 3 as compared to Group 4 is thus shown to be due to the stimulating action of gonadotropic hormone upon the testes

EXPERIMENT 42

Pregnancy Test in Rats

This test is based on the excretion. During pregnancy, of chorionic anterior pituitary like (C. A. P. L.) hormone. Its presence is shown by the reaction of the ovaries of immature rats.

Material and Equipment

Urine from a pregnant woman, Specimen of ordinary (non-pregnant) urine.

Procedure

1. Both urine preparations are extracted with ether and the discarded (some urine samples are toxic, the toxic substances being ether soluble). The urine samples are then filtered and kept in the refrigerator.
2. Four immature female (21-24 days old) rats are taken, two are injected s.c. with each of the urine samples. The injection schedule is 2 injections daily of 0.5 c.c. per injection for 3 days.
3. The animals are sacrifice at the end of 100 hours. after the first injection and the reproductive organs of the two groups are contrasted.

EXPERIMENT 43

Anti-fertility Test in Female Rats

Anti-fertility action in the female may result out of the following :

(i) inhibition of ovulation ;

(ii) prevention of fertilization;

(iii) interference of transport and / or implantation of fertilized ovum; and

(iv) destruction and resorption of the early implanted embryos.

Material and Equipment

Microscope, Test drug.

Procedure

1. Adult female rats of established fertility (having produced two consecutive litters) are examined on seven consecutive days by microscopical observation of vaginal smear.
2. Anti-fertility test drug is administered to the female rats and are matched in pair with males of proven fertility.
3. The females are examined for the following :
    (a) Sign of mating as indicated by the presence of sperm in vagina ; prolongation of the average time from pairing to the first insemination is indicative of anti-fertility effect

    (b) estrus cycle changes by vaginal smear examination ;

    (c) inspection of uterus for number of implants ;

    (d) number of litters at birth ; and resorption of fetuses revealed by the difference between (c) and (d).

EXPERIMENT 44

Anti-fertility Test in Male Rats

In the males there are two possible mechanisms by which an anti-fertility agent may act :

(i) Suppression of spermatogenesis at any of the stages resulting in sterility, associated with oligospermia or aspermia

(ii) a quantitative changes in spermatozoa rendering them nonfunctioning.

Material and Equipment

Same as the female sterility test.

Procedure

1. Fertile adult male rats are taken for anti-fertility test.
2. Males are treated with anti-fertility drug and are mated each with two females of known fertility.
3. And following examinations are carried out:
   (a) Sign of mating as indicated by the presence of sperm in vagina of females : Calculation of the date of insemination from the date of birth (gestation period approximately 21 days) permits an estimate of the duration of sterility; pseudopregnancy (presence of leucocytes in vaginal smear for 10-14 days) is indication of aspermic copulation.
   (b) normal estrus cycle is indicative of failure to mate due to an effect on libido; and
   (c) motility test of sperm from base of epididymis in males.

EXPERIMENT 45

Anabolic Androgenic Test in Rats

Androgens effect changes in the male sex organs and result in anabolic effect as well. Thus teststerone causes an increase in weight of the seminal vescles and produces retention of nitrogen. Since most compounds that show one effect also show the other. Moreover, it is desirable to find compound that shows only one effect, other being conspicuously absent. For the myotrophic (anabolic) effect the gain in the weight of the levator ani-muscle ; for the ardrogenic effect, the gain in weight of ventral prostate gland is measured.

Material and Equipment

Surgical instrument, Test drug, Weighing machine,

Procedure

1. Male rats of a single strain, 21 days old are castrated and are maintained on a diet and tap water ad *libitum.*
2. Groups of 5 or more animals are used. Each animal is given daily s. c. injections of the test drug in oil vehicle for 7 days, begining with the day of castration. Control group will only receive oil vehicle.
3. On the 8th day, 22 to 26 hrs. after the last injection, the animals are killed.
4. Dessection of the levator ani muscle is effected after removal of skin in the scoroal area between the base of the penis and the anus. The posterior aspect of the perineal complex is cleared from fat and connective tissues with forceps, particular care being taken to disclose the contraction at either end of the lavator where it joins the bulbocavernosus muscle. The rectum is transected just caudal to point where the levator loops around it dorsally. The body of the levator-ani is then freed of the rectum and is removed by incission at the points of attachment to the bulbocavernosus muscle. The levator ani is cleaned of any connective tissue and weighed to the nearest 0 1 mg The ventral prostate gland is also weighed.
5. The ratio of the weight gain of the levator-ani (the muscle weight of treated animal minus the mean muscle weight of the control group) to the weight gain of the ventral prostate gland is cafculated.

EXPERIMENT 46

General Directions for Blood Pressure Experiments in Rats

Material and Equipment

Duble-membrane tambour, Ink-writing recorder, Calibration manometer, Kymograph.

[Because of the extremely rapid rate of the rat's heart 250-350 beats per minute) and the lag of the mercury column, recordings of the blood pressure made by use of the mercury manometer are unsatisfactory. Such a record is shown, and it will be noted that the individual pulse beat is barely visible. No magnification of the thrust of the mercury column is possible, and, in addition, one must use a sooted kymograph drum, which is inconvenient and messy. Much better records are obtained with the special tambour and ink-writing devices which are described.

Procedure

1. Both chambers of the tambour are filled with saline, making sure no air bubbles are present, and the pen is attached and tested for smooth, uninterrupted writing.
2. The kymograph drum is to be calibrated. For this a mercury manmeter is attached to the tambour, and, by means of a syringe, saline is forced into both systems, the pressure being indicated by the mercury column. A pressure of 100 mm. is introduced into the lower tambour, with the upper stopcock open. This stopcock is then closed, and the drum is revolved. Additional pressure, in increments of 25 mm. is then introduced, and the drum is revolved for each. Pressure is then released to 100 mm., the tambour clamped off, and the mercury manometer removed. From now on, the setup must not be disturbed until it is used, or the calibration will not be accurate.
3. After the anaesthetic has taken effect, the rat is fastened to a frogboard, either with clips or, better, with strips of adhesive tape. Routinely, the trachea is cannulated first, to avoid respiratory difficulties later; ether may be administered, if necessary, by holding a tuft of cotton over the open end of the cannula. The carotid is now cannulated, heparin administered. other necessary surgery performed, and the carotid cannula finally attached to the tambour.

EXPERIMENT 47

Determination of the Cardiac Output in Rats

The cardiac output can be calculated from the oxygen consumption and the arteriovenous oxygen difference by application of the Fick principle. The oxygen consumption is determined by direct measurement with a recording microspirometer. Arterial blood samples are obtained by cannulation of the carotid artery, and mixed venous blood is obtained by introducing a cardiac cannula directly into the heart. The blood samples are analyzed for their oxygen content, using micromethod of Scholander.

The cardiac output is influenced by a number of factors, including drugs such as adrenalin, acetylcholine, nitrites, etc. In this experiment the effect of adrenalin on the cardiac output is demonstrated.

Material and Equipment

Instruments for cannulation, Heart cannula.

(18-gauge needle about 4 cm. long, which has previously been marked at the proper depth of introduction, using a rat cadaver).

Oxygen consumption apparatus, Kymograph, Stop watch, Scholander Roughton analyzer, Caprylic alcohol.

Procedure

The oxygen consumption apparatus ia set up.

1. Wick is soaked in 20% NaOH and inserted in the absorption tube. The water jacket is filled with water at room temperature or just below.
2. With the absorption tube attached to the microspirometer, the apparatus is calibrated by drawing lines around the kymograph drum at 5 c.c. intervals.
3. The microspirometer and absorption tube are filled with oxygen.
4. The trachea and left carotid artery are cannulated ; 0.25 c. c. heparin is injected
5. The cardiac cannula is introduced into the right external jugular vein, through the superior vena cave and into the right auricle. The end of the cannula is moved up and down with each heart beat.

6. The arterial and cardiac cannula are connected to the tubes mounted in the suport which is clamped to the animal board. 1 c.c. syringes are connected to each of the tubes.
7. The rubber tube is attached from the absorption apparatus to the trachea of the animal. The writing needle rose and fell with each respiration but also showed a fall due to oxygen consumption. When the needle just crosses one of the calibration lines, the stop watch is started. Then samples of arterial and mixed venous blood are withdrawn while oxygen consumption is being determined. After the samples have been obtained, the time and temperature are recorded just as the needle crosses one of the other calibration lines.
8. The blood samples are stored anaerobically in the 1 c'c. syringes by plugging the tips of the syringes with round toothpicks, If the analysis for blood oxygen is not to be completed immediately, the samples should be stored in the refrigerator.
9. 0.005 mg/kg. of adrenalin in injected i, v. and the cardiac output is determined immediately as above.

EXPERIMENT 48

Determination of Blood Volume in Rats

Material and Equipment

Vital red dye (0 5%), Heparin,

Instruments for carotid cannulation, Calorimeter, Centrifuge.

Procedure

[Two rats are necessary for the determination. One is called the control'; it merely supplies the plasma used in preparing the standard solution. The other is the 'experimental animal', which is to be injected with the dye solution. Its weight must be known to determine the amount of dye to be injected.

The quantity of dye to be injected is arrived at by a rough estimation of the animal's plasma volume. Repeated experiments have set the total blood volume of the rat at about 6% of the body weight. If a rat weights 300 gms., the blood volume will be about 18 c.c. and the plasma volume about 9 c.c. The figure will be used in making up the standard solution. For the dye injection, 1 c.c. per kilogram is given, or 0.3 c.c. for a 300 gms. rat.

1. Cannulation of the carotid artery is done in control rat.
2. Injection is made into the artery, by means of a 1 c.c. syringe, directly through the cannula an amount of saline equal to the volume of dye which will be injected into the experimental animal, plus 0.25 c. c, of heparin. Mix the fluid remaining in the cannula with blood by repeatedly withdrawing about 0.5 c.c of blood into the syringe and then forcing it back.
3. Replacing the 1 c.c. syringe by a 10 c.c one and, after about 3 minutes, as much blood as possible, as rapidly as possible – at least 5 c.c. is withdrawn directly placed in a centrifuge tube. The blood is carefully handled to avoid haemolysis,
4. Canulation of the carotid artery of the experimental animal is done in the same manner.
5. Injection of 0.25 c.c. of heparin plus the calculated amount of dye (1 c.c./kg) is done and mixed as before. It is noted that the total amount: of fluid injected into each animal is the same. After 3

minutes. as much blood as possible is withdrawn and placed carefully in a centrifuge tube. From this the relative volume of cells and plasma is determined.

6. Both samples are kept in the centrifuge for 30 minutes.
7. While the samples are in the centrifuge, the standard solution is prepared. The standard solution is made by adding the amount of dye injected to a volume of saline equal to the calculated plasma volume. That is, a 300 gms. rat would have an estimated plasma volume of 9 c.c, and would have been injected with 0.3 c. c. of the dye. The standard solution would then be 9 c.c. of saline plus 0.3 c. c. of dye.

   The colorimeter is prepared by adjusting each vernier to read zero when the cup is raised to rest against the bottom of the plunger. Both cups are then filled with the stand and solution and set at 20 mm., and the light source is adjusted to give a uniform field. Standard solution is discarded from the right hand cup and it is replaced with the unknown solution.
8. The samples from the centrifuge are removed and the level of plasma and cells are marked. The plasma of the control should be clear, that of the experimental animal should be stained pink.
9. 2 c.c, of plasma is taken from the experimental sample and 6 c.c. of saline is added to it. From the control 2 c.c. of plasma plus 2 c.c. of the standard solution plus 4 c.c. of saline are used. The plasma from the control gives the standard solution the same degree of turbidity, when examined in the colorimeter, as that of the experimental solution. Syringes are the most convenient means of measuring.

   The two solutions are compared in the colorimeter. Proportions of blood cells and plasma are determined. The amount of water required to fill the tube to the level of the red cells and from there to the top level of the plasma are measured from a syringe.

EXPERIMENT 49

Effects of Thyroidectomy and of Thyroxin on the Basal Metabolic Rate in Rats

In this experiment the normal B.M.R. of a group of rats is determined. They are then subjected to thyroidectomy, and, after an interval of several weeks, the B.M.R. determination is repeated. Thyroxin is then administered, and its ability to return the B.M.R. to (or above) the normal is demonstrated.

Material and Equipment

Apparatus for determination of oxygen consumption, Sterile pack and surgical instruments, Thyroid preparation (a preparation containing 20 mg, purified thyroxine per tablet is satisfactory)

Procedure

To determine the oxygen consumption, the apparatus is first caiibrated.

1. The desiccator is filled with a 5% sodium hydroxide solution (at room temperature) to just below the level of the cage in which the rat is placed, and a flask having about the same volume as the rat is placed in the cage,
2. With the tambour and writing lever adjusted, 20 c.c. of air are forced into the desiccator, and a line is run around the drum.
3. Then 40 c.c. of air is withdrawn, and another line is drawn.
4. The flask is now removed and filled with water at 40°C and replaced in the cage. By means of a thermometer graduated in tenths of a degree, the volume equivalent of the rise in pressure, per degree rise in temperature, is determined. This correction is necessary in calculating the oxygen consumption.
5. The rat is now placed in the chamber, 25 - 30 c.c. of air is forced in, and the drum is started. As the carbon dioxide is absorbed, the line which is being written on the drum falls.
6. At the instant it crosses the upper calibration line, a stop watch is started and the temperature noted. When the lower calibration line is crossed, the time and temperature are again recorded. This provides the data for the calculation of oxygen consumption. The determination is repeated as the rat moves out. In any case three close checks on each animal should be obtained.

Thyroidectomy

1. Prepare for an aseptic operation as previously described.
2. Make a ventral mid-line incision through the skin of the neck, push the salivary glands to one side, and expose the trachea by slitting the overlying muscle in the mid-line. The thyroid is the reddish, bi-lobed structure lying on either side of the trachea just below the larynx. The parathyroids may be seen as tiny, whitish bodies at the tip of the upper lobe. An effort should be made to leave them behind ; in any case, however, calcium gluconate should be added to the drinking water for several days after the operation to avoid parathyroid tetany.
3. A small bridge of thyroid tissue (the isthmus) connects the two lobes across the trachea. With fine forceps divide the isthmus and, holding onto one end, dissect carefully underneath the lobe. Two structures must be watched for the inferior thyroid artery, which is the main blood supply to the thyroid (the superior is smaller and may be disregarded), and the recurrent laryngeal nerve, which lies close to the trachea and passes below the lobe of the thyroid. The artery must be either ligated or clamped off with the tips of a fine hemostat; the nerve must not be disturbed at all, or respiratory difficulties will develop later, and the animal may die. With these precautions in mind, the lobe is dissected free, leaving a small amount at the upper tip enclosing the parathyroid, and removed.
4. The other lobe is then removed in the same manner.
5. Close the wound with fine silk sutures through the muscle and two or three more through the subcutaneous tissue.
6. Close the skin incision with wound clips. Watch the animals for a few days for signs of respiratory distress and give them a 1 % solution of calcium gluconate for drinking water.
7. After several weeks (it requires from 2 to 4 weeks for symptoms of hypothyroidism to become pronounced! the oxygen consumption is again determined as described above. A considerable fall (20-40%) will have occurred.

   Thyroidectomized animals are more sensitive to thyroxin than normal animals ; therefore, these same rats are now used to demonstrate its action.
8. Crush a tablet of thyroxine in saline and inject, s. c., a dose of 1 mg/kg. Redetermine the oxygen consumption 48-72 hours. later. The oxygen consumption will be normal or somewhat above.

EXPERIMENT 50

Determination of Oxygen Consumption, Respiratory Quotient and Basal Metabolic Rate in Rats

In this experiment the amount of oxygen consumed and the amount of carbon dioxide produced, per minute of time, are determined. From these figures the respiratory quotient is calculated. and the basal metabolic rate namely, the calories of heat produced per square meter of body surface per hour, is determined.

Material and Equipment

1(N) Sodium hydroxide solution, 30 % sodium hydrosulfite solution, Apparatus for collecting expired air, Van Slyke manometric apparatus, 50 c. c. syringe.

Procedure

1. The trachea is cannulated and valve system is attached to trachea and collecting bulb. The collecting bulb is equipped with a three way stopcock.
2. About 100 c. c. of air is collected and discarded through the other outlet of stopcock. This is for the purpose of washing atmospheric air out of the tubes.
3. Now time is measured accurately for collection of 100-150 c. c. air. This is the air used for analysis and must consist of only expired air; it is therefore important to maintain a slight positive pressure against the valves to prevent leakage.

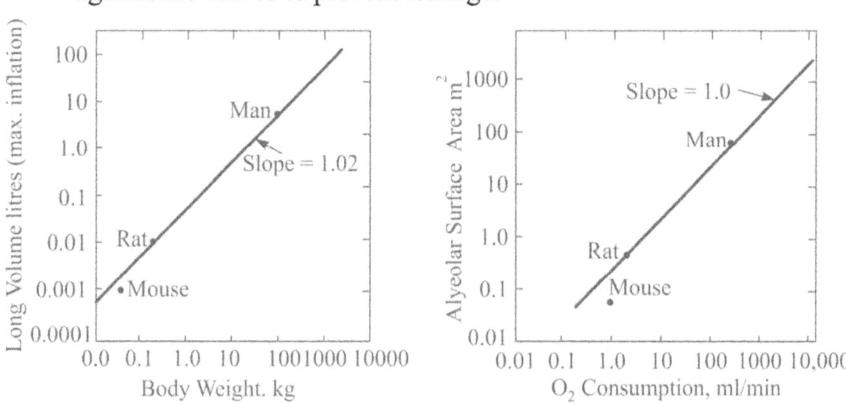

Fig. 22 Comparative study of Oxygen Consumtion of Mouse, Rat and Man.

4. A short rubber tube is attached to one of the stopcock outlets and the tube and the outlet are filled with light mineral oil. The plunger of the 50 c. c. syringe is also oiled, The syringe is attached to the rubber tube and about 50 c. c. of the expired air is withdrawn.

5. The rubber tube is removed along with the syringe, and to it short piece of capillary tube is attached, the end of which is fitted with a rubber collar. The syringe will contain some oil which can be used to fill the capillary tube. The sample is now ready for intro duction into the Van Slyke.

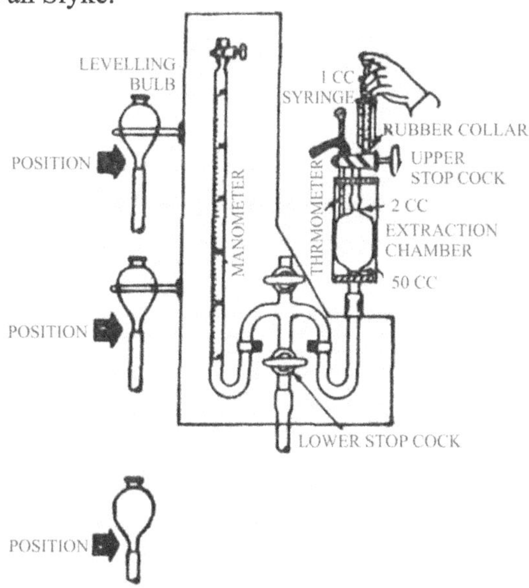

Fig. 23 Van Slyke manometric apparatus.

6. With the bulb in position 1, the mercury is permitted to flow slowly upward through the upper stopcock and into the chamber until the chamber contains 1 or 2 c. c.
7. The surface of the mercury is dried with a filter paper. Leaving some mercury in the chamber and stopcock to serve as a seal, the remainder is drawn down to slightly below the 50 c. c. mark below the bulb.
8. Placing level of bulb in position 2 and the mercury is brought exactly to the 50 c. c mark, pressure is read.
9. With leveling bulb in position 2 and lower stopcock open, about 35c.c, of the expired air sample is introduced by holding the

rubber-tipped end of the capillary tube tightly against the flare of the chamber above the stopcock. The excess oil is removed by exerting pressure on the plunger and forcing it out below the mercury before opening the stopcock. The stopcock is made open and the air entered.

10. Again the mercury is taken down to the 50 c. c, mark and the pressure is read. Temperature is also recorded.
11. By means of a 1 c. c. syringe, exactly 1 c. c, of 1 (N) sodium hydroxide solution is introduced The mercury is raised until it fills approximately the lower third of the bulb, and is shaken for 2 minutes.
12. Lowering below the 50 c.c. mark and bringing the mercury meniscus (not the solution) exactly to the 50 c.c. mark, the pressure is read.
13. 3 c.c. of the 30% hydro sulphite solution is admitted in the same manner, it is shaken for 3 minutes with the mercury about one-third up the bulb, bringing down to the 50 c. c. mark and with the mercury meniscus on the mark, the pressure is read.
14. Now the remaining gases are ejected from the chamber without loss of solution. The mercury meniscus is brought down to the 50 c.c. mark and the pressure is read.
15. The solution is ejected and the apparatus is cleaned. Calculation is done according to Peters & Van slyke method.

EXPERIMENT 51

Respiratory Rate, Tidal Air and Pulmonary Ventilation of Rats

Material and Equipment

Pair of one-way valves, Collecting bulbs, Stop watch.

Procedure

1. A rat is anaesthetized and the trachea is cannulated.
2. With the values, the outlet valve is connected to one of the collecting bulbs, maintaining a slight positive pressure (about 1 cm. of water, against the valve to prevent leakage. As air collects, the other bulb is lowered, maintaining the positive pressure. When the water in the collecting bulb reaches the upper calibration, the stop watch is started. The respiration rate is counted which is easiest done by watching the inflow of air through the trap, and 100 cc. of air is collected.

EXPERIMENT 52

The Ileum of the Mouse

Local anaeasthetics, Analgesics, and substances, having activity like quinidine, may owe their essential qualities to their active opposition of acetylcholine.

Material and Equipment

Tyrode solution, Atropine, Apparatus for isolated preparation, Acetylcholine chloride, Test drug.

Procedure

1. Four different strips of mouse ileum are used.
2. To the bath fluid in which the strip of ileum is suspended is added acetylcholine chloride, so that the concentration stands as 0.2 μg/ml of the bath fluid.
3. Later to 1 minute a solution of drug is added. A geometric series of drug concentrations, commencing with 10^{-9} M, are given until the acetylcholine contraction is done away with.
4. The bath solution is washed out repeated times after a test, and the strip is stayed at rest for a fixed interval between the tests. The determination of the highest inactive concentration of the compound is achieved and then the concentrations that are twofold and fivefold of this are given.
5. At least four doses of atropine, in concentration between 5.6×10^{-9} M and $5\ 6 \times 10^{-9}$ M are added to the bath between the doses of test compound, and thus the drug Can be estimated to have some % of activity of atropine.

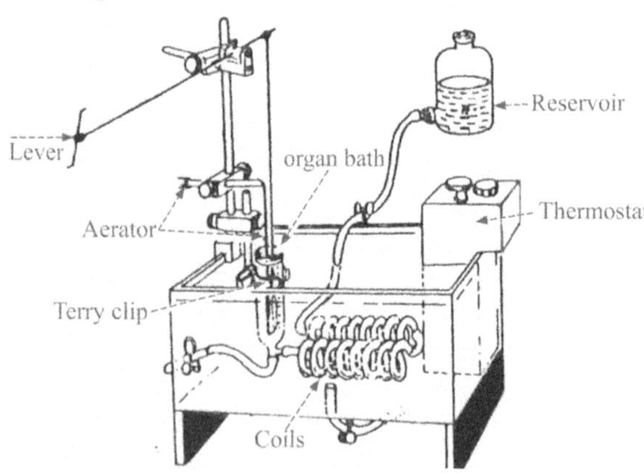

Fig. 24 Apparatus for isolated preparation

EXPERIMENT 53

Anococcygeus Muscle Preparation of Rat

The two anococcygeus muscles in rat crop up from upper coccygeal vertebra behind the terminal colon, pass ventrocaudally to pass rapidly over the lateral side of the colon and unit in front of colon a few milimeter from the anus to constitute a ventral band. Histamine lacks in effectiveness almost in this preparation. A prohibitory response to field stimulation is obtained after the administration of drug guanethidine.

Material and Equipment

Apparatus used for isolated preparation, Test drug, Tyroid solution, Surgical instruments.

Procedure

1. Killing of a pale rat is effected by a blow on the head and it bled,
2. The abdomen is opened in the mid line, the pelvic split and the bladder and urethra removed adopting precautions to prevent damage of the belly band of muscle lying ventral to the colon.
3. The colon is then cut through at the pelvic brim, the lower part of the abdomen portion pulled forward and the connective tissues cleaned until the anococcygeus muscles come to light for apparent vision.
4. The muscles are isolated, if necessary with the extrinsic nerves intact. The band of the belly is cut through and each muscle is mounted in a 10 ml. bath containing Tyroid solution at 37°C. Response of test drug is recorded.

EXPERIMENT 54

Fundus Strip of the Rat

This preparation is in fact, very sensitive to several agents, and therefore, may be utilised to test for compounds, similar to any one of them, and for their antagonists. It is useful for assay test of serotonin, histamine amphetamine sulphate, bradykinin, barium chloride, ATP, acetylcholine etc.

Material and Equipment

Kreb's solution, Apparatus for isolated preparation, Test drug, Surgical instruments.

Procedure

1. After hit on the head and exsanguination, the rat is opened and the stomach cut out and dropped into the bath solution. The antrum is cut transversely and then the fundus is cut to preserve the logitudinal muscle and to provide a strip. After a strip is tied to the ends, the strip is gently expanded and fringes of pyloric tissue are trimmed off. One end is tied to tissue holder and lowered into the organ bath, the thread tied to the other end is attached to the liver.

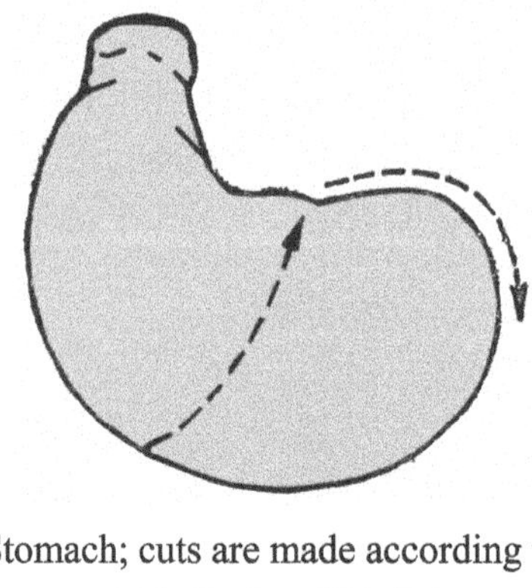

Fig. 25 The Stomach; cuts are made according to arrow mark.

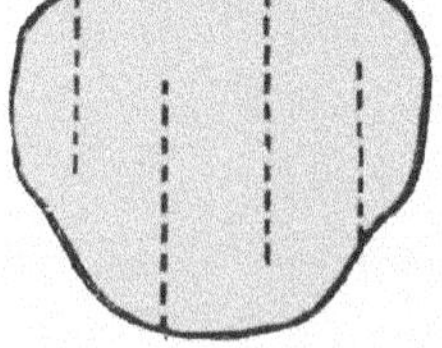

Fig. 26 Cuts are made in this sheet of muscle so as to produce a strip.

2. The bath is 0.85 cm in diameter and 15 cm. deep with the tissue holder and aeration tube is placed, the bath hold 5 ml. If the strip is unattended to for more than 5 minutes. the bath solution is allowed to flow lowly, otherwise the strip shortens.
3. The bath is aerated with 95% osygen + 5% carbondioxide and contains Kreb's solution at 37°C.
4. The liver is arranged to enlarge the contraction by 16 times.

   A constant load of 1 gm. is coupled with a light spring, so that as muscle contracts, the restoring capacity increases. A spring of 3 cm. extending 3.2 cm. per gm. of load is attached to the lever at a point twice the distance of the muscle from the fulcum, A vibrator reduces the friction of writing point. Replacement of spring-lever can also be made by pendulum lever.
5. During the cycle, the drug is added to the bath, after 90 secs. the bath is washed out by overflow. A weight is added to the lever so that it comes to rest on a bar. This operation expands the muscle to an uniform degree. After a fixed interval, 15 to 30 secs.

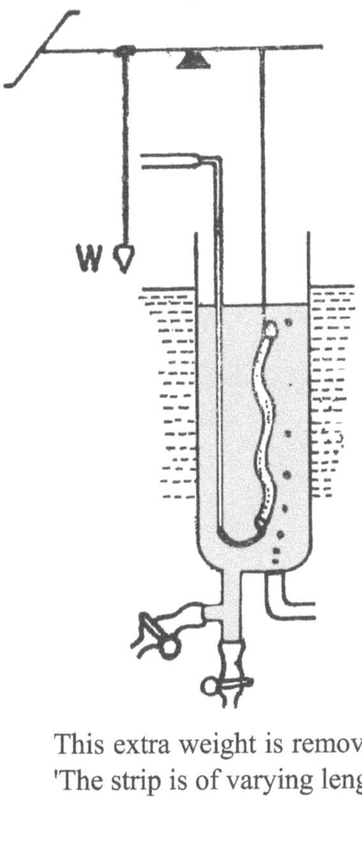

Fig. 27 The organ bath containing Kreb's solution, oxygen (95%) + carbondioxide (5%) at 37°C. Extra weight, W, used for stretching the preparation.

This extra weight is removed, After 2 minutes. the cycle starts again 'The strip is of varying length in course of use from 6 to 12 cm.

EXPERIMENT 55

The Duodenum of the Rat

This preparation stands on different phase from almost all others employing isolated organs in which the relaxation rather than the contraction is measured. It is useful for detecting and estimating kinins, of which those that have been studied chemically are peptides. Application of actylcholine and serotonin results in contractions. Vasopressin and oxytocin cause relaxation when present in large doses.

Material and Equipment

De Jalon's solution, Atropine, Test drug, Instrument for isolated preparation, Surgical instruments.

Procedure

1. The proximal 3 cm. of duodenum from a rat weighing 150 to 250 gms is suspended in a 10 to 15 ml. bath containing atropinized (1 mg/ml.) De Jalon's solution at 30° to 31°C.
2. The tissue is stored at 4° to 6°C for 2 to 3 hours. before use, since this storage affect the deportment of the tissue favourably.
3. The act of magnifying by 15 times is used with the writing lever, whose tension is 0.5 gm. for most duodenal strips, The dose cycle is 3 to 4 minutes. with 30 seconds. of contact time. The bath is washed out by upward displacement and overflow.

EXPERIMENT 56

The Ileum of the Rat

Material and equipment

De Jalon's solution, Atropine, Apparatus for isolated preparation Surgical instruments.

Procedure

1. A segment of 3 cm. from the terminal ileum of a starved rat, weighing 150-250 gms. is suspended in a tissue bath of 2 ml. in volume.
2. The nutrient solution is that of De Jalon's solution at 31°C atropinized with 1 mg/ml.
3. A dose cycle of 5 to 10 minutes. is used, looking tinto the rapidity of the response.
4. The test substance is allowed to act for 40-90 secs,

EXPERIMENT 57

The Jejunum of the Rat

This test is useful in the analytical screening for muscarinic activity, The rat Jejunum has the advantage over the guineapig ileum in that, it gives only insignificant responses to ganglionic instigation such as nicotine.

Material and Equipment

Tyrode solution, Apparatus for isolated preparation. Test drug, Surgical instruments,

Procedure

1. A piece of Jejunum about 2 cm, in length is taken from decapitated rat and washed in Tyrode solution. It is suspended in the usual manner in a bath containing 10 ml. of Tyrode solution through which air is bubbled at 37°C.
2. The response to addition to muscarinic agents are recorded on a smoked drum with the aid of writing lever.

In this preparation the response to acetylcholine or another standard is altered with the response to the test substance.

EXPERIMENT 58

The Seminal Vesicle of the Rat

This preparation has the advantage over guidence pig seminal vesicle, of being not susceptible to histamine.

Material and Equipment

Modified Ringer-Locke solution, Apparatus for isolated preparation, Test drug. Surgical instruments.

1. The seminal vesicles of rats are removed and suspended in modified Ringer-Locke solution.
2. First, the coagulation glands are carefully taken out without injury to the vesicles. After removal of extraneous tissue, the vesicles, are transected distal to their point of entrance in the ductus deferens.
3. A 15 ml. tissue chamber is used for two vesicles. The temperature is 37.5°C. The chamber is aerated with 95% oxygen +5% Carbon-dioxide, and Ringer-Locke solution is allowed to flow in at the rate of 100 ml/min. Flow is hindered when drugs are added.
4. Ten minutes. after the vesicles are placed in the chamber, doses of 90 mg. epinephrine, at 6 minutes. intervals produce regular response.
5. With a view to testing sympathetic drugs, epinephrine is given until regular responses are achieved, Then 6 minutes. Following the last dose, the test substance is allowed to act for 1 minute. in chamber and dose of epinephrine is then repeated. Two further doses are given 6 and 12 minutes. later,

EXPERIMENT 59

The Colon of the Rat

Material and Equipment

De Jalon's solution, Apparatus for isolated preparation, Test drug, Surgical instruments.

Procedure

1. A. segment of ascending colon, 3 cm. long is removed from a rat weighing 150 to 250 gms.
2. It is suspended in a tissue bath, 2 ml, in volume. In de Jalon's solution at 25°C the spontaneous activity lessens below that found at higher temperatures, but it may still cause trouble.
3. The dose cycle is 3 or 4 minutes., with 40-60 seconds, of contact time.

EXPERIMENT 60

The Uterus of Rat

The responses obtained with this tissue are quicker than those produced by the fundus but slower than those produced by the ileum in that there is often a latent period before anything appears to happen. The sensitivity of the uterus depends upon its condition. For this experiment the rat should be young, between 120 -150 gms. in weight, and in estrus. It may be necessary to bring it into estrus by injecting s.c. 24 hours, beforehand, a dose of stilboestrol (0.1 mg/kg. body weight).

Material and Equipment

De Jalon's solution, Apparatus for isolated preparation, surgical instruments, Test drug, stilboestrol,

Procedure

1. The animal is killed and the abdomen opened. The intestine is pulled aside or removed, so as to expose the two horns of the uterus.
2. The mesenteric attachments are cut away and the two horns are transferred to a dish containing de Jalon's solution.

   The two horns are cut open longitudinally, so that the preparation is a sheet of muscle, instead of a narrow tube. It is usually satisfactory to divide each born further longitudinally and so obtain 4 pieces from one animal.

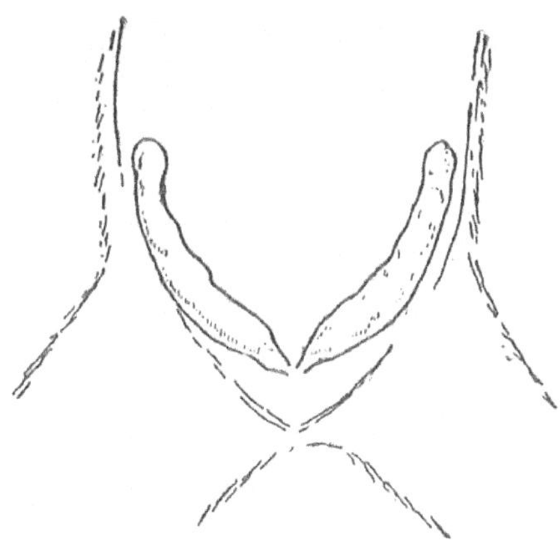

Fig. 28 Two horns of the uterus.

3. One thread is attached at each and of each piece and the preparation is mounted in de Jalon's solution which is aerated with oxygen (95%) and carbondioxide (5%). One thread is attached to a fixed pin and the others to a lever fitted with a frontal-writing point. The load on the lever is about 0.5 gms. and magnification about 5-fold. The bath should be 5-8 cm, long with a volume of about 10 ml, The temperature is usually between 30 minutes and 32°C. The preparation usually takes 15-30 minutes, to settle down before regular responses are obtained.

4. Text drug is added to the bath and waited for $1\frac{1}{2}$ minutes, to get proper response.

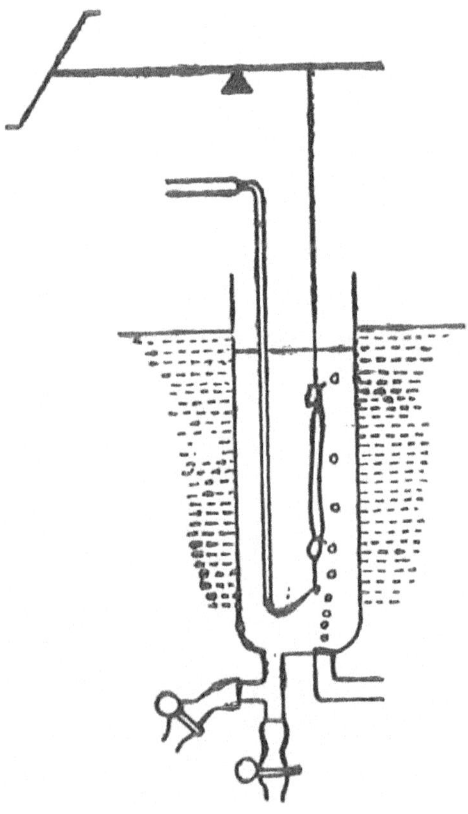

Fig. 29 De Jalon's Solution ; Oxygen (95%) + Carbondioxide (5%) 30°c.

EXPERIMENT 61

Test for Diuretic Activity in Rats

The Lipschitz model has been proved to be a standard method and widely used for screening of potential diuretics.

Material and Equipment

Metabolic cage, male wistar rats, urea, 0.9% NaCl solution

Method used (Lipschitz Test)

Method for testing diuretic activity in rats has been firstly described by Lipschitz et al. (1943). Water and sodium excreted by the test animals can be compared to rats group treated with a high dose of urea. The "Lipschitz- value" is the quotient between excretion by test animals and excretion by the urea control.

Lipschitz value = excretion by test animals/excretion by the urea control

Procedure

1. Male Wistar rats (100–200 g) were taken.
2. Three animals in each group were kept in metabolic cages having a wire mesh bottom and a funnel to collect the urine. Stainless-steel sieves are placed in the funnel to retain feces and to allow the urine to pass.
3. Standard diet (Altromin® pellets) and water ad libitum is given to rats.
4. Fifteen hours before the experiment food and water are withdrawn.
5. Two groups of three animals are used for one dose of the test compound for the purpose of screening. The test compound (50 mg/kg in 0.05 ml water/kg body weight) is administered orally.
6. Two groups of three animals were administered orally 1 g/kg urea.
7. In addition to this, 5 ml of 0.9% NaCl solution per 100 g body weight are given by gavage.
8. Urine excretion is recorded every 5 and after 24 h. The sodium concentration or content of the urine is determined by flame photometry. Active compounds are tested again with lower doses.

9. Urine volume excreted per 100 g body weight is calculated for each group. Results are expressed as the "Lipschitz-value" i.e. L.V=T/U, where, T is the response of the test compound, U, urea response.
10. L.V value of 1.0 and greator than this means a positive effect. Potent diuretics, give Lipschitz values of 2.0 and more.
11. Calculation is made for 24 h excretion period as well as for 5 h indicates the duration of the diuretic effect. Similar to urine volume, quotients can be calculated for sodium excretion.
12. Dose-response curves can be established using various doses.
13. In case of hydrochlorthiazide dose is (0.1-1.6 mg/kg) in 25 ml/kg 0.9% NaCl solution.

EXPERIMENT 62

Test for Anticonvulsant Activity in Mice

This study has been used to evaluate antiepileptic drug. PTZ (metrazol) is CNS stimulant and induces convulsion against which the antiepileptic activity has to be observed.

Materials and Equipments

Swiss albino mice, PTZ, plastic cages

Procedure

1. Swiss albino Mice (18-22 g) were used and the test compound or the reference drug is injected sc. or i.p. or sometimes given orally to groups of 10 mice.
2. Another group of 10 mice were taken as control group.
3. 15 min after sc.-injection, 30 min after i.p.-injection, and 60 min after oral administration MTZ (Metrazol), 60 mg/kg injected subcutaneously and then each animal is placed into an individual plastic cage and observation was done up to 1 hour.
4. Seizures and tonic-clonic convulsions are recorded. At least 80% of the animals in the control group have to show convulsions.
5. Number of protected animals in treated group is calculated as the percentage of affected animals in the control group.
6. Calculation of ED50-values is done. Furthermore, the time interval between MTZ-injection and occurrence of seizures can be measured.
7. The delay of onset is calculated in comparison with the control group.
8. Doses of the antiepileptic drugs, Chlordiazepoxide (20 mg/kg i.p.), diphenylhydantoin (10 mg/kg i.p.) and phenobarbitone sodium (20 mg/ kg i.p.) were found to be effective.

EXPERIMENT 63

Hypolipidemic Activity in Rat

Hyperlipidemia, or hyperlipidaemia involves abnormally elevated levels of any or all lipids and/or lipoproteins in the blood. It is the most common form of dyslipidemia High fat induced model has been employed for assessment of lipid lowering activity of hypolipidemic drugs in rat.

Materials and Equipments

Cholesterol rich diet, plastic cages, wistar rat of either sex (male or female)

Procedure

1. Male wistar rats were taken into study and were housed in plastic cages (four to five animals in each cage) with sawdust bed.
2. Three groups were made at least 6 animals in each group. First group is supplied with the diet and solvent (PEG 400) i.e. control group and group second is supplied with cholesterol rich diet.
3. Group third receive cholesterol rich diet and drug gemfibrozil (100 mg/kg/day) is administered orally up to 25 days to the third group.
4. At the end of the treatment, rats were fasted for 12 hrs, anaesthetized with chloroform by inhalation in anaesthetic chamber. Blood is collected in collecting tubes from the animals of each group i.e. control as well as the groups that receives cholesterol rich diet and group that receives cholesterol rich diet and gemfibrozil both via cardiac puncture.
5. Estimation of various lipids like HDL, LDL, triglyceride and total cholesterol can be done with the use of cholesterol reagents, HDL, LDL, triglycerides kits and taking absorbance (cholesterol, HDL, triglyceride at 505 nm) by using U.V spectrophotometer.

   Formulae used

   Cholesterol conc. (mg/dl) = abs of test /abs of standard × 200

   HDL conc. (mg/dl) = abs of test /abs of standard × 50

   Triglyceride= abs of test /abs of standard × 200

   LDL = total cholesterol – triglyceride/5-HDL

6. Concentrations in mg/dl of cholesterol, HDL, LDL, triglycerides were obtained from all the blood samples of control group, group that receives cholesterol rich diet and group that receive cholesterol rich diet and gemfibrozil both and finally the comparison is made via statistical analysis.
7. Similarly, hypolipidemic activity of another hypolipidemic drugs can also be assessed.

EXPERIMENT 64

Antitumor Activity in Mice by using Ehrlich Ascites Carcinoma (EAC) Cell line

EAC is one of the commonest tumors; it is widely used in induction of liquid tumor in mice because of shorter life span, rapid proliferation and 100% malignancy. Ascites liquid is gray-white, or sometimes has a light bloody viscous liquid and contains 10 million neoplastic cells in 0.1 cc (Akta, 1996; Kaleolu and li, 1977). Transplantation of EAC cell line by i.m route in leg muscle also induces solid tumor.

Materials and Equipment

EAC cell line, neubers chamber for counting, saline phosphate buffer, microscope, trypan blue dye.

Procedure

1. Swiss albino mice (18 -22 g) were used
2. Two groups were made 12 animals in each group
3. First group is transplanted with EAC cells (2×10^6 cell/mouse through i.p) and no drug is given to this group.
4. Last group is transplanted with EAC cells and after 24 hrs drug (5-flurouracil 20 mg/kg/day or bleomycin 0.3 mg/kg/day) administered at alternate days orally for 14 days.
5. EAC cell can be preserved during course of study by transplanting 2×10^6 cells/mouse i.p into fresh mouse after every 9 day from the previous mice bearing cell line
6. After 24 hrs of the last dose six animals of each group is sacrificed by cervical dislocation for the evaluation of anticancer activity by studying several parameters such as tumor weight , tumor volume, viable and non viable tumor cell count
7. Rest six animals of each group were left as such and supplies with standard diet and water ad libitum for study of the parameters such as median survival time (MST) and percent increase in life span.
8. Weight of the mice was recorded before and after the sacrifice, and difference in weight gives the tumor weight. For tumor volume the ascetic fluid is withdrawn from the peritoneal cavity and volume is measured in graduated centrifuges tube.

9. Counting of cancer cell is done by the use of neuber's chamber by diluting the 0.1 ml tumor fluid 100 times by phosphate saline buffer and 1 drop of this is placed on the neuber'slide and counting is done same as WBC counting.
10. Viable and non viable cell count can be determined by staining with trypan blue dye non viable cells take the stain and appear as blue where as viable cell do not.
11. From the rest six animals of each group survival studies were done by evaluating mean survival time (MST) and %increase in life span (% ILS)

    Mean survival time = [1st Death + Last Death] / 2
12. Calculation of % ILS is done by using formulae

    ILS (%) = [(Mean survival of treated group/ Mean survival of control group) – 1] x100
13. The MST and % ILS are the two main parameters for the assessment of potency of any anticancer drug.
14. Finally the comparison of all above parameter is done between the EAC control (no drug treatment) and group bearing EAC cell line that receive 5-Flurouracil and Bleomycin.

EXPERIMENT 65

Test for Respiratory Depressant Drug effect in Rats

It is a non-invasive method for distinguishing central from peripheral nervous system effects of respiratory depressant drug.

Materials and Eqiupments

Male spague dawley rats, plastic cages, plethysmograph, sodium cyanide

Procedure

1. Male Sprague Dawley rats (270-490 g) are taken for study. In the study rats are exposed to the gas and sodium cyanide gas mixtures using a two chambered plethysmograph.
2. The body of the animal is enclosed in one chamber which is used to measure ventilator parameters, while the head is enclosed in a cylindrical plastic head piece which is attached to the body chamber. A rubber collar around the neck of the animal is used for the separation of the two chambers.
3. From compressed gas tanks specified gaseous mixtures are delivered to the head chamber at a rate of 2 l/min. The type of gas mixture is controlled by a multi-port stainless steel manifold with individual valve controls. The gas mixture contains either normal breathing air (21% O_2, 79% N_2) or elevated CO_2 (8% CO_2, 21% O_2, and 71% N_2).
4. The animals are first exposed to the normal air mixture for 5-10 min and then subjected to the elevated CO_2 mixture for 5 min. The mean value for the 5 min CO_2 exposure is calculated for each ventilator parameter.
5. Following CO_2 exposure, rats are exposed to normal air mixture for a period of 5 in or until the ventilator parameters return to normal before sodium cyanide is injected. Sodium cyanide (300 μg/kg) is administered as a bolus i.v. injection using a catheter implanted into a tail vein. The peak change in each ventilatory parameter is measured during the 1-2 min period of ventilator stimulation following sodium cyanide injection.
6. For carotid body denervation, the rats are anesthetized with a cocktail containing ketamine (26.9 mg/kg), xylazine (2.9 mg/kg) and acepromazine (0.3 mg/kg).

7. Incision in the the middle of the neck is made and the glossopharyngeal nerve on each side of the neck is isolated. Using a dissecting microscope, the glossopharyngeal nerve is cut cranial to the carotid sinus nerve. The rats are allowed to recover 4–7 days prior to use. Changes in ventilatory parameters are measured in conscious restrained rats using a body plethysmograph chamber with an internal volume of 2.2 l that seals around the neck of the animal and encloses the body within the chamber. Airflow rates within the chamber are measured using a pneumotach port and a differential pressure transducer attached to the plethysmograph chamber.
8. The pressure signal is analyzed using an Upper Airway Monitor (Buxco Electronics. Inc., Sharon, CT) and values for tidal volume, respiratory rate, minute volume, peak expiratory flow, inspiratory time and expiratory time are determined for each breath. Average values of these parameters are calculated and expressed as digital output every 0.1 min using an analog-digital convertor.
9. Mean inspiratory flow (respiratory drive) is calculated by dividing tidal volume by inspiratory time, while fractional inspiratory time is calculated by dividing inspiratory time by the sum of inspiratory and expiratory times. Continuous tracings of flow and volume changes are also recorded to evaluate qualitative changes in ventilatory patterns.
10. Mean values of treated groups are considered to be statistically different from the control group if the calculated P value is < 0.05.

EXPERIMENT 66

Wound Healing Activity in Rats by Excision Wound Model

Wound healing is a fundamental response to tissue injury that results in tissue integrity, which is due to the synthesis of the connective tissue matrix. Collagen is a major protein of the extracellular matrix and is the component that ultimately contributes to the wound strength.

Material and Equipment

Swiss wistar strain rats, framycetin sulphate, polypropylene cages, ether as anaesthetic.

Procedure

1. wistar strain rats (150-200 g) were used .
2. Rats were anaesthetized by using little concentration of ether.
3. A circular wound of 500 sq mm is made on depilated ethanol sterilized dorsal thoracic region of rats (excision wound model as described by Morton and Malone).
4. Two groups of the animals were made on which receive no treatment i.e. control group and group second receive framycetin sulphate cream (FSC) i.e standard group.
5. Framycetin cream is applied to the standard group once a daily during course of experiment.
6. Two parameters were studied, wound closure and epethelisation time the wounds were traced on mm^2graph paper on 3, 6, 9, 12, 15, and 18 and thereafter on alternate days until the healing is complete. The percentage of wound closure was calculated.
7. The period of epithelisation was calculated as the number of days required for falling of the dead tissue remnants of the wound without any residual raw wound.
8. Finally the comparison is done between control and standard group.

EXPERIMENT 67

Antiparkinson Activity in Rats

Materials and Equipments

Male albino rats, phenothiazine, polypropylene cages.

It is a extrapiramidal disorder characterized by the hyperkinesia, rigidity and tremor. Parkinson induction is done by phenothiazines against which antiparkinson activity of drug is noted. The detection of the antiparkinson activity through the screening for parasympatholytic activity is indirect.

4 Stages of catatonia induced by phenothiazines (Wirth et al). These stages were determined by the test at the 2, 4, 6, and 22 hours after s.c injection of phenotrhiazine

Stage 1: Animal shows no movement, sits quietly on its place; light push to animal cause some movements.

Stage 2: Same as stage 1 but light push to animal shows no movement.

Stage 3: Animal makes posture for e.g. when its forelegs placed on a cork of 3 cm high.

Stage 4: Animals maintains its fixed position, while sitting on the hind legs, one of the forelegs if placed on a cork of 9 cm high, and other foreleg is allowed to hang free.

Procedure

Method

1. Male albino rats (300 g) given 5 mg/kg phenothiazines intraperitoneally. That produces catatonic response; parasympatholytic drugs effective in Parkinsonism antagonize the catatonic responses.
2. Now the rats are placed on the table one of the front paw on a cork of 3 cm high (stage3) and then on a cork of 9 cm (stage 4).
3. A Positive Catatonic reaction means failure to correct the imposed posture in 10 seconds.

4. Stages are tested on left and right side both. Half point is given to the positive response shown by stage 3 and 1 point is given to stage 4. The maximal catatonic response is 3 points. At each dose level, a group of 4 animals is used.
5. Test compound is injected i.p 15 minute before the perphenazine and finally percent inhibition of catatonia is calculated against a group of rats injected only with perphenazine.
6. Drugs which inhibited perphenazine at a dose of 2 mg/kg are atropine, scopolamine, trihexyphenidyl, benzotropine and biperiden.

EXPERIMENT 68

Test for Antishock Agents in Rats

Agents which have the ability of the adrenergic and ganglionic blockade inhibit the development of irreversible shock. The sympatholytic drugs may be screened for antishock activity. Traumatic shock by Noble and Collip (1942) method is induced in rats by tumbling the rats inside the rotating the drum having two shelves.

Materials and Equipments

Female albino rats, revolving circular drums, bretylium tosylate

Procedure

1. Female albino rats (135-175 gm) are used. In each experimental run up, a control group animal is placed in one drum, where as a drug-treated animal is placed in the other. The revolving circular drums are identical to each other, and are rotated on the same axial shaft so that the rates are same for treated and control group animals
2. Drug is given 18-24 hours before trauma, animals those remain alive for 48 hours after being subjected to trauma are considered as permanent survivors. All animals are fasted 24 hrs prior to drumming.
3. Drums were rotated at 40 revolutions per minute for 10 minutes, 50 percent mortality is seen in male rats and female shows less mortality than rats. At 700 revolutions the mortality is 100% for male rats and 75 % mortality is seen in female rats.
4. Drugs are dissolved in saline and are administered i.p in a volume of 0.3 to 0.5 ml, control group receive same amount of saline and the mortality results are analysed statistically with the help of chi-square test and Yates'correction. It is observed that the % mortality gets diminished in case of test group when compared with the control group.
5. Guanethedine sulfate (10 mg/kg) and bretylium tosylate (10 mg/kg) can be used for above experiment for the detection of antishock activity in rats. They act by inhibiting the release of catecholamines.

EXPERIMENT 69

Test for Hepatotoxicity in Mice

Organic compounds such as haloalkanes have been supposed to be hepatotoxic, it is a matter of interest to know whether the pharmacologically active compound is hepatotoxic or not. Screening is done on the factor that the damaged liver prolongs the effect of drug.

Materials and Equipment

Male swiss albino mice, olive oil, pentobarbital

Procedure

1. Mice weighing (20-30 gm) is taken for the study, they are provided with a solution of the test substance in olive oil subcutaneously. The volume deposition is 0.05 ml/10 gm of body weight. In case of water solube substances propylene glycol is a preferable vehicle.
2. Twenty four hours later, 45 mg/kg of pentobarbital sodium is administered intraperitoneally. The mean sleeping time of pentobarbital is 9.0 ± 7.3 minutes for the control mice, and if it increases to 23 minutes then it would be a significantly prolonged. The $ED_{50,}$ for increased sleeping time can be determined with the use of groups of mice, given various doses of the test substances.
3. Another test is done to confirm, by using second drug, bromsulfalein (100 mg/kg) is given i.v, after the administration of fifteen minute 0.5 ml of blood is taken via cardiac puncture using light ether anesthesia, if the plasma conc. is found to be greator than 5.8 mg/100 ml is taken as significant, and shows hepatotoxicity.

EXPERIMENT 70

Antiemetic Activity in Wistar Rats

Vomiting is supposed to occur by the stimulation of the chemoreceptor trigger zone (CTZ), morphine and apomorphine are drugs that stimulates this zone.

Materials and Equipment

Male wistar rats, apomorphine hydrochloride, plastic cages

Procedure

1. Male wistar rats were taken for the study kept in cages having shavings woods and an observation window.
2. Test drug is given subcutaneously and after one hr of the test drug apomorphine hydrochloride (1.25 mg/kg) is administerd intravenously. Now, after the 5, 10 and 20 minutes animals were kept under observation by the person who is unaware of treatment.
3. Now, the zwangsnagen or compulsory gnawing is observed, absence of gnawing is direct indication of antiemetic activity.

INSTRUMENTS USED FOR MICE AND RATS EXPERIMENTS

Surgical Instruments, Injections and Cannula used in Laboratory Mice and Rats Experiments

Instruments

The choice and selection of instruments depends very much on personal taste and trial but the following instruments are likely to be imperative.

Medium-sized scissors with either straight or curved blades are useful for cutting the skin and soft tissues of small animals and for cutting coarser sutures. *Blunt-ended scissors* are convenient for blunt dissection. 5 inch length scissors, straight and curved or flat are deemed appropriate.

Fine scissors should only be used for cutting fine blood vessels, e.g. the rat carotid artery and femoral artery. Some *fine scissors* have the blades set at an angle to the handles; this allows the points to be kept up, which is an advantage when cutting connective tissue around vessels. And for cutting fine blood vessels or the dura matter, *spring action capsular scissors* are suitable.

Large forceps are needed for general work: 6 inch broad, fluted dissecting forceps are suitable. Some people find *large toothed forceps* as convenient for ensuring a firm grip of skin or large masses of tissue but they may tear. ***Dissecting forceps,*** 6 inch, *2* ×3 teeth are suitable.

Medium-sized fine toothed forceps are ideal for ensuring a firm grip of smaller pieces of connective tissue or muscle and for holding the cut end of the trachea open. *Irish forceps,* straight fluted grip, fine tooth 1:2 are suitable.

Medium-sized fine curved forceps are used for delicate blunt dissection, e.g. beneath the trachea of the rat or around vessels blood in most animals, and for passing ligatures. *Irish forceps,* fluted grip, fully curved, are suitable.

Medium-sized fine straight forceps are needed for delicate blunt dissection. $3\frac{1}{2}$ inch ophthalmic dissecting forceps are suitable.

Fine pointed forceps are needed for picking up fine sutures, holding open or dilating cut blood vessels, and for stripping connective tissues from small blood vessels and nerves. *Watchmakers forceps,* No. 4, are suitable.

Large haemostatic forceps, with straight or curved points, are required for clamping large blood vessels in the animals or tissue masses containing bleeding vessels. 6 inch artery forceps, with either straight or curved points, are suitable. They should have box joints to ensure a firm grip,

Medium sized haemostatic forceps, with straight or curvep points, are useful for clamping small blood vessels, 5 inch straight and curved *artery-forceps* are suitable.

Both *large and medium artery forceps* have ratchets so the pressure between the ends can be properly adjusted.

Small haemostatic forceps, with straight or curved points ('bull-dogs') are needed for the temporary occlusion of blood vessels. *Artery forceps* (straight or curved) are suitable. The 2 cm, size is used for rats

Needle-holding forceps are required for ensuring a firm grip on curved suture needles.

A fine blunt seeker is very useful for holding open cut blood vessels to aid the insertion of a cannula.

A large scalpel with No. 20 disposable blade is useful for cutting skin quickly and cleanly.

A medium-shed scalpel with blade No. 10 is useful for cutting small areas of skin and cutting open the trachea,

Cannula

Successful cannulation depends upon having cannula of the right size and shape. For insertion into the trachea, glass cannula are particularly suitable because they are transparent and also because they can easily be cleaned. For arteries and veins much finer cannula are needed and it is easier to make these out of plastic than out of glass. Polyethylene or nylon tubing is drawn out in a very small flame. The technique used is similar to that for glass except that these plastics soften at much lower temperatures.

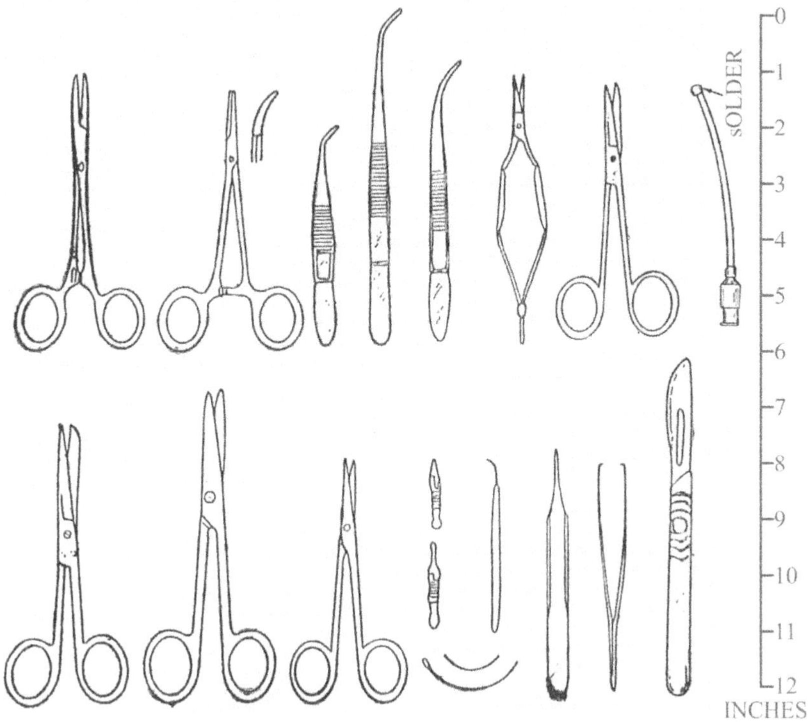

Fig. 30 Instruments used for mice and rate experiments.

The two materials behave differently and nylon is easier to work. After practice, cannula can be made with tips as small as 0.25 mm. The nylon cannula are stiffer than the others and consequently, less likely to collapse when the vessel is tied onto them.

Fine plastic tubing is particularly useful since it makes it possible to place the injection block at a convenient distance from the site of the injection, so that there is no risk of dislodging the cannula, The dead space is extremely small, even with several centimetres of, for example, 0.9 mm. internal diameter tubing. This can be inserted directly into the femoral or cephalic, though it must be pulled down to about 0.25 to 0.5 mm. at the tip before it can be inserted into the femoral vein of the rat.

TRACHEAL

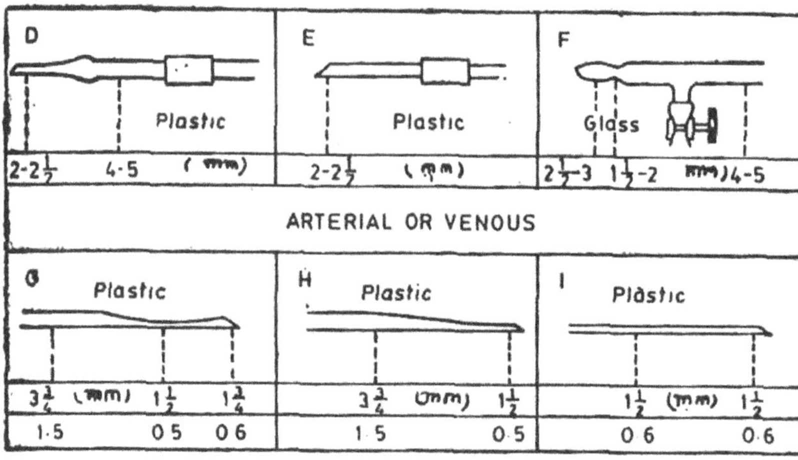

Fig. 31 Details of Cannula used for rat.

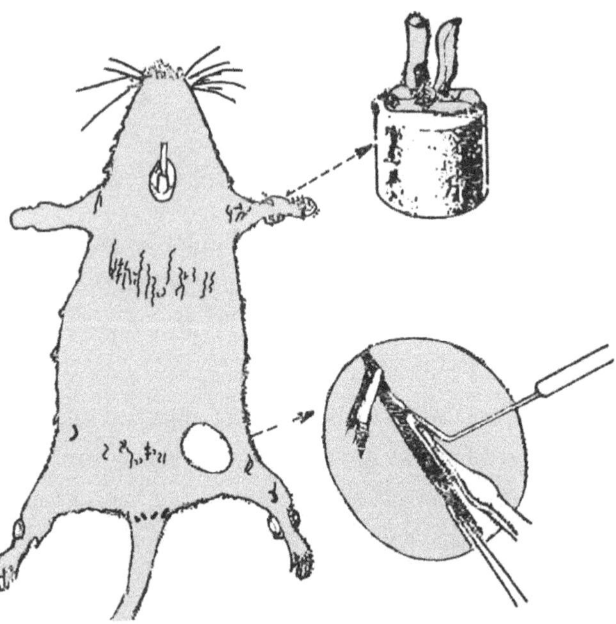

Fig. 32 Cannulation to rat.

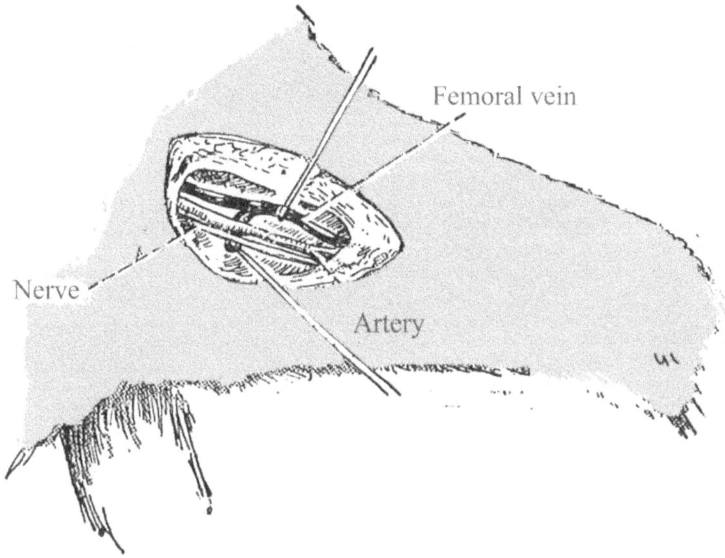

Fig. 33 Venous Cannulation of rat; a, location of femoral vein; b, procedure.

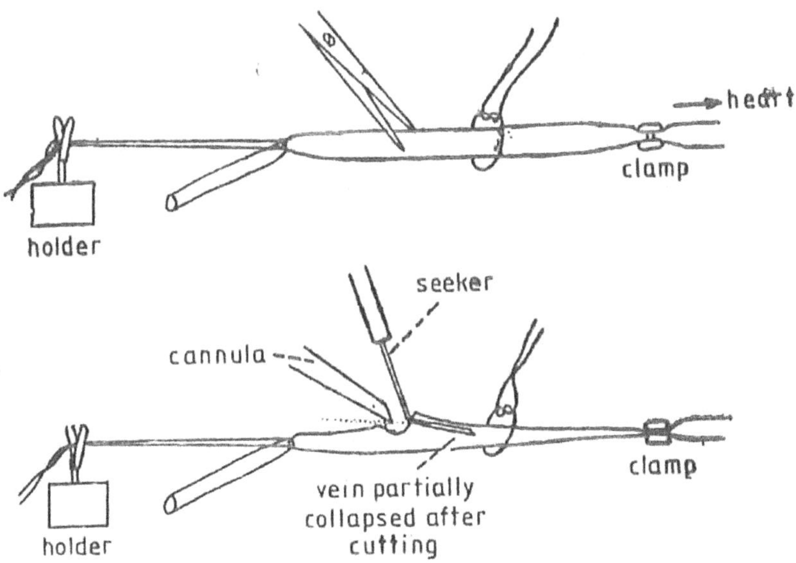

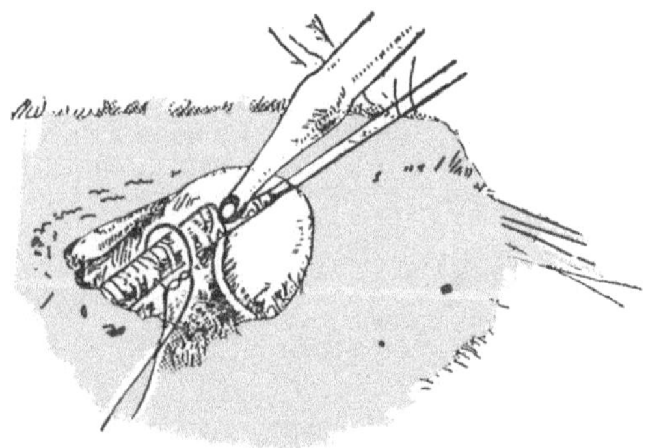

Fig. 34 Tracheal cannulation to rat.

Injections

For any injection during animal experiments the needle must be sharp and of suitable size (Table) Even if it need not be sterile, there is no justification for re-using it if it is at all blunt, because disposable needles are not expensive. Disposable syringes, too, are cheap and much more robust than glass ones. Though it is just possible that some drugs may dissolve slightly in the plastic, this does not usually necessitate using glass ones. In many experiments sterility does not matter, and syringes, as opposed to needles, may be re-used many times, especially if they are being used always for the same drug solution. In these circumstances an appreciable saving in expense is made by re-using 'disposable' plastic syringes. These can even be used for different drugs provided they are well washed. A few drugs are reputedly particularly difficult to wash out and it is probably wisest to use a fresh syringe. for example, with secondary or tertiary bases, but with quaternary salts the useful life of a syringe can be very long, being limited only by the tendency for the graduation to become worn away. This can be reduced by placing transparent tape over the graduation.

Table

		I.V.	**I.P.**	**S.C.**	**I.M.**	**P.O,**
Mouse	Needle size Max dose/volume	27 G $\frac{1}{2}$ in. 0.4 ml	25 G $\frac{3}{4}$ in 1ml,	25 G $\frac{3}{4}$ in.0.4ml.	25 G $\frac{3}{4}$ in.0.4ml.	18 G 2 in 1 ml.
Rat	Needle size Max.	–	25 G 1 in,	25 G 1 in	25 G 1 in.	–
	Max. dose/volume	–	2 ml.	1 ml.	0.4 ml.	–

DRUG DOSES USED ON LABORATORY MICE AND RATS

Table 1 Drug Doses used on Laboratory Mice and Rats

Drugs	Animals	Dose per kg body weight and route	Effects & Remarks
A	B	C	D
Acetylcholine chloride (keep the soln. at pH 4, stock soln. is made up in 5% $NaHPO_4$ soln.)	Rat	1 to 10 μg i. v.	Muscarinic (nicotinic in high) agonist
Adrenaline bitartrate (Soln. last only for hrs.)	Rat	3 μg i.v.	Adrenoceptor agonist
Alloxan monohydrate	Rat Mouse	50 mg i.v. 150 mg i.p. 80 mg i.v.	Produces experimental diabetes mellitus 1 week before experiment 24 hours experiment 3 days before experiment
Aminooxyacetic acid	Rat	20 mg i.p.	Increases central GABA level : 60 min prior to test.
d-Amphetamine sulphate (Soln. last for weeks)	Rat	3 to 5 mg s.c. 0.7 mg s.c.	CNS stimulant and anorectic : Increase locomotor activity.
Apomorphine HCl (Soln. last for weeks add ascorbic acid)	Rat Mouse	0.2 to 0.8 mg s.c. 0.1 to 1.0 mg i.p.	Dopaminergic agonist
Aspirin (solid last for weeks, suspended in 1% CMC)	Rat	200 mg p.o.	To induce gastric ulcers
Atropine methylnitrate	Rat Mouse	2.5 to 5 mg s.c. 2 to 5 mg i.p.	Peripheral muscarinic receptor blocker
Atropine sulphate	Rat Mouse	1 mg i.v. 2 to 10 mg i.p.	Muscarinic receptor blocker
Baclofen HCl	Mouse	1 mg i.p.	GABA antagonist
Benserazide HCl	Rat	50 mg i.p. 3 times at 2 hourly intervals. 200 mg i.p. 3 times at 2 hourly intervals.	In lower doses only peripheral depletion of DOPA decarboxylase both central and peripheral noradrenaline (NA) depletion in high doses.

Table 1 *Contd...*

Drugs	Animals	Dose per kg body weight and route	Effects & Remarks
A	B	C	D
	Mouse	50 mg i.p.	min. before experiment.
Bretylium tosylate	Rat	5 to 20 mg i. v.	Adrenergic neuron blocker : 2 hr. prior to test
Bromocriptine mesylate	Rat	1 to 5 mg s.c.	Dopaminergic agonist
Carbachol chloride (Soln. last for hrs., keep at pH4)	Rat	0.2 to 0.5 μg, i.v.	Gastric acid stimulation
Carbon tetra-chloride	Rat	0.1 to 1 ml p.o. total dose	Induction of liver damage
Carrageenin	Rat	0.1 ml of 1% soln., subplantar	Phlogistin
DL-p-Chlorophenyla lamine (PCA)	Mouse	5 mg i.p.	5HT depletory : 24 hr. before experiment
p-Chlorophenyla lamine (PCA)	Rat	300 mg daily for 3 days i.p.	5-HT depletory; results in 80% depletion of 5-HT and much less of NA and dopamine (DA).
Store at 0°C, before use it is dissolved in 1 (N) NacH at pH 8.9)	Rat	100 mg every 48 hr for 5 5 days s.c.	
	Mouse	150 to 300 mg 12 hourly for 3 days i.p.	
DL-p Chlorophenylalamine methylester HCl	Rat	100 mg daily for 4 days i.p. 150 to 300 mg daily for 3 day i.p.	Soluble from of PCPA to be stored at 0°C. Experiment to be done 12 hr. after the last dose.
Cimetidine	Rat	100 mg i.p.	H_2 – Receptor blocker
Cinanserin HCl	Rat Mouse	100 mg i.p. 5 mg i.p.	5-HT blocker : 30 min. prior to test

Table 1 *Contd...*

Drugs	Animals	Dose per kg body weight and route	Effects & Remarks
A	B	C	D
Cocaine HCl	Mouse	4 mg i.p.	Locomotor activity by DA uptake inhibition.
Cromoglycate or cromolyn sodium	Rat	2.5 to 5 mg × 2 for 4 days p.o.	Mast cell stabilizer
Cyproheptadine	Rat	50 μg s.c	5-HT and histamine blocker
Deoxycorticosterone acetate (DOCA)	Rat	25 mg × 2 tab. s.c. implantation	Produces hypertension in unilateral nephrectomized rat
		5 mg s.c. twice a week × 7 weeks	Drinking water replaced by 0.9% NaCl after 5 to 6 weeks.
Destmethylimi pramine (Desipramine)	Rat Mouse	0.1 to 0.5 mg i.v. 25 mg i.p. 0.2 20 mg i.p.	Neuronal uptake inhibitor of CA ; 1 hr. before experiment
Diethyldithio carbomate sodium (DDC)	Mouse	500 mg i.p. followed after 2 hr. by 500 mg s.c.	Brain NA depletion by 46% 6 hr after s.c. administration DA is increased and 5-HT remains unchanged
Diethylstiboestrol (Stillboestrol)	Rat	1 mg i.p/I m. 0.1 mg i.m/s.c.	24 hr. prior to experiment for priming young female rats
Dihydroergotamine tartrate	Rat	0.5 mg i.v.	α – Adrenergic blocker
Dipyridamole	Rat	10 mg i.v.	Phosphodiesterase inhibitor
Dissulfiram (Tetraethylthiuram disulfide) (sns[emded with tragacanth)	Rat	100 mg i.p.	NA Systhesis inhibitor (dopamine β oxidase and aldehyde dehydrogenase inhibitor)
Domperidone HCl	Rat	0.1 to 2 mg i.p.	Peripheral DA antagonist
L-DOPA HCl	Rat Mouse	100 mg i.p.	Dopaminergic agonist (to alter motor activity)
Eserine salicylate (Soln. is made in acidulated saline)	Rat Mouse	0.25 mg i.p. 0.1 mg s.c.	Anticholinesterase, 20 min. before experiment
Evans blue	Rat	20 to 40 mg i.v.	1 to 2% aq. soln. injected 5 min. before experiment

Table 1 *Contd...*

Drugs	Animals	Dose per kg body weight and route	Effects & Remarks
A	B	C	D
Femoxetin	Rat	2.5 to 10 mg i.p.	5-HT neuronal uptake inhibitor
Fenfluramine HCl	Rat	15 mg p.o. 5 to 10 mg s.c./i.p	Anorexigeric agent; 5-HT depletor; depletes 5 HT by 50% ; release NA by 4%, DA by 3% 24 hr. after administration
FLA-63 (dissolve in hot dilute tartaric acid)	Rat Mouse	25 to 50 mg i.p. 40 to 50 mg i.p,	NA synthesis blocker (dopamine-hydroxylase inhibitor) without affecting DA and 5 HT stores; action within 2 to 5 hr.
Fluoxetine	Rat	75 to 10 μg total i.c.v. 3 mg p.o.	5-HT uptake inhibitor (central effect); 30 min before experiment.
Formalin	Rat	0.1 mg of 2% soln. under aponeurosis	Phlogistogen; repeated after 48 hrs.
Guanethidine sulphate	Rat	1 to 5 mg i.v.	Adrenergic neuron blocker ; 6 hrs before experiment.
Haloperidol [dissolve in PG : Ethanol (60 : 40)]	Rat Mouse	0.5 to 5 mg i.p. 0.5 to 2.5 mg i.p.	DA antagonist
Heparin sodium (soln. last for weeks when kept below 25°C)	Rat	20 mg i.v.	Anticoagulant
Hexamethonium bromide (soln. last for weeks)	Rat	10 to 20 mg i.v.	Ganglion blocker
Histamine dihydrochloride or acid phosphate (soln. last for hrs ; keep at pH 4)	Rat	0.25 to 1 mg i.v. total dose	Bronchospasm
Hyaluronidase	Rat	A total dose of 0.4 ml of 600 IU/ml in saline s. c. on the dorsum of the foot	For testing anti-inflammatory agents
Hydrocortisone	Rat	10 to 40 mg s. c.	Anti-inflammatory agent

Table 1 *Contd...*

Drugs	Animals	Dose per kg body weight and route	Effects & Remarks
A	B	C	D
6-Hydroxydopamine (6-OHDA) HBr (store at 0°C, dissolve in cold 0.9% NaOH containing ascorbic acid)	Rat	250 μg i. c. v. in 25 μl 50 mg i.v. (2 doses of this within 24 hrs. followed a week later by 2 × 100 mg dose)	Experiment to be performed 24 hr. after but within 1 week after the last dose.
		150 mg × 14 days s. c. 50 mg × 2 i. p. on day 1 : 100 mg × 2 i.p. from day 2 to 4	Start experiment on day 5 or 6 day.
6-Hydroxydopamine (6-OHDA) HCl	Mouse (newborn)	50 mg × 2 doses followed 8 days later by a single dose of 100 mg i.v.	24 hrs. after the 3rd dose the animal is killed
5-Hydroxytryptophan (5-HTP) methylester	Rat Mouse	2 to 25 mg i.p. 25 to 50 mg i.p.	Precursor of 5-HT tested 30 mins. after administration
Hyoscine HBr (soln. last for days)	Rat Mouse	0.05 to 1 mg s.c. 0.5 to 4 mg s.c.	Muscarinic blockers; 15 mins. Before experiment
Imipramine HCl	Rat Mouse	20 mg. i.p. 50 to 100 mg i.p.	Neuronal uptake blocker of CA.
Indomethacin (dissolve in 0.3% $NAHCO_3$ soln.)	Rat	4 to 5 mg i.p.	Anti-inflammatory agent
Iproniazid phosphate Isoprenaline HCl (soln. last for hrs. keep the soln. at pH4 add ascorbic acid)	Rat Rat	50 mg i p. 50 to 500 μg s.c,	MAO inhibitor 24 hrs. before experiment to inducmyocardial necrosis
Kainic acid (dissolve in 0.5 mM phosphate buffer)	Rat	1 to 10 μg i.c.v.	Neurotoxic to GABA ergic neurons
Leptazol (soln. last for weeks)	Rat	70 to 112 mg i.p./s.c. 0.2 ml of 6% solution total i.v.	Convulsant
Lithium chloride	Rat Mouse	150 mg i.p. 40 to 300 mg i.p.	Produces behavioral changes (head twitches)
Mephenesin	Rat	80 mg i. m.	Strychnine antagonism and inhibition of polysynaptic reflexes

Table 1 *Contd...*

Drugs	Animals	Dose per kg body weight and route	Effects & Remarks
A	B	C	D
Mepyramine maleate	Rat Mouse	5 to 10 mg. i.p, 2.5 to 25 mg i.p.	H_1-Receptor blocker
Metergolin (suspend in 5% CMC)	Rat	0.5 mg i.p.	5-HT antagonist; 1 to 2 hrs. prior to experiment.
Methacholine chloride	Rat	Total dose of 5 to 10 μg i.v.	Gastric acid stimulant
α–Methyldopa hydrazine	Rat	200 mg i.m.	Dopa decarboxylase inhibitor ; depletion of peripheral NA stores
α–Methyl-paratyrosine HCl (α-MPT)	Rat	150 mg i.v. 200 mg i.p. 100 mg s.c. 30 to 50 mg i.c.v	Tyrosin hydroxylase inhibitor producing NA and D.A. depletion maximal depletion of CA occurs 12 hrs. after the administration;
	Mouse	100 to 200 mg i.p.	Administration 16 to 18 hrs before experiment.
α–Methylparatyrosine methylester HCl (soln. in prepared in 0.5 M phosphate buffer saline (pH 7.4), and store at 0°C)	Rat Mouse	150 to 250 mg i.p. 100 to 250 mg i.p.	CA synthesis blocker Depletion occurs maximum by 4 hrs
Methysergide bimaleate	Rat Mouse	20 mg i.p. 1 to 5 mg i.v.	5-HT antagonist; 30 min. before experiment
Metiamide	Rat	25 to 100 mg ip.	H_2-Receptor blocker;
	Mouse	25 to 200 μg total i.c,v.	30 min prior to experiment
Metoclopramide dihydrochloride	Rat	10 to 50 mg i.p.	Selective DA antagonist ; to induce catalepsy or stereotyped behavior
Metoprolol tartrate	Rat	0.2 to 5 mg s.c.	Selective – adrenoceptor blocker
Mianserin HCl	Rat	13 mg i. p.	5-HT blocker: 30 min prior to experiment
Morphine sulphate or HCl (soln. last for weeks)	Rat Mouse	1.5 to 10 mg s.c. 1 to 5 mg. i.m.	Analagesic
Muscimol	Rat Mouse	10 to 30 mg i.p. 50 to 200 mg total i. c.v. 3 mg i.p,	GABA agonist ; 30 mins, prior to test
Nalorphine HCl (soln. last for weeks)	Rat Mouse	5 mg i.p. 1 to 5 mg i.p.	Opioid antagonist with partial agonist activity

Table 1 *Contd...*

Drugs	Animals	Dose per kg body weight and route	Effects & Remarks
A	B	C	D
Phenylephrine HCl	Rat	5 to 70 μg i.v. total dose	α-Adrenoceptor agoint
Phenylquinone	Mouse	0.25 ml. i.p. (0.02% in 5% alcohol)	Production of writhing syndrome for evaluating analgesics
Phenytoin	Rat	135 mg i.p. 300 mg s.c.	Anticonvulsant
Pimozide (dissolve in 0.1% tartaric acid and pH adjusted to 5.5)	Rat Mouse	10 mg i.p. 1 mg i.p.	DA blocker; 3 hr. before experiment
Piperoxan HCl	Rat Mouse	20 mg i.p. 10 to 20 mg i.p.	α-Adrenoceptor blocker: 10 min to 1 hr. before experiment
Prazosin HCl	Rat Mouse	0.1 to 1 mg i.v. 1 mg i.p. 20 mg i.p.	α–Adrenoceptor blocker; 15 min to 1 hr. before experiment
Propranolol HCl (soln. last for hrs. keep at pH4)	Rat Mouse	15 mg i.p. 5 mg s.c. 1 mg i.v. 5 to 10 mg i.p.	– Adrenoceptor blocker; 4 hrs, before experiment1 hr. before experiment
Quipazine maleate	Mouse	3 mg i.p.	5-HT agonist
Reserpine (soln. lasts for days, add in 10% ascorbic acid and pH is adjusted to 4.8)	Rat Mouse	1 mg i.v. 1 mg i.p.	For cardiovascular effects
	Rat	1 mg i.m.	For behavioral effects; 15 hrs. prior to experiment.
	Rat	0.5 mg i.p. × 14 days 5 to 15 mg i.p./s.c.	
	Mouse	5 mg i.p.	
Salbutamol sulphate	Rat	0.5 to 5 mg i.p.	Selective 2-adrenoceptor agonist
SKF-525A	Rat	40 mg i.p.	Hepatic microsomal enzyme inhibitor

Table 1 *Contd...*

Drugs	Animals	Dose per kg body weight and route	Effects & Remark
A	B	C	D
Naloxone HCl	Rat Mouse	0.1 to 1 mg s.c.	Opiate antagonist
	Mouse	1 to 5 mg i.p.	Precipitation of morphine withdrawal
Neostigmine bromide (soln. last for weeks)	Rat Mouse	0.1 to 1 mg s.c./i.v. 0.2 0.1 mg s.c.	Cholinesterase inhibit
Nicotine acid tartrate (soln. last for weeks)	Rat	0.1 mg i.v.	Ganglion stimulant : higher than 0.3 mg dos produces convulsion
Nifedipine (dissolve in 30% ethanol)	Rat	5 to 50 μg i.v.	Calcium antagonist: blocks calcium channel
Niludipine Nisoldipine (dissolve in 5% PG)	Rat	50 μg i.v.	Calcium antagonists
Noradrenaline bitartrate of HCl (Add 1% ascorbic acid to minimize oxidation of soln)	Rat	3 μg i.v.	α-Adrenoceptor agonist
Oestradiol valerate or benzoate (dissolve in ethanol : Saline (3.7)	Rat	0.1 to 1 mg s.c.	Administered 1 day before experiment
Oxotremorine (Soln. last for weeks)	Rat Mouse	0.2 to 0.4 mg i.p. 0.5 to 2 mg i.p. 2 mg i.p.	Tremorogenic
Oxymeta-zoline HCl	Rat	0.3 to 3 μg i.v.	α-Adrenoceptor agonist
Pargyline HCl	Rat Mouse	50 mg i.m. 75 mg p.p.	MAO – inhibitor ; 3 hrs. before experiment
Pethidine HCl (soln. last for days)	Rat	30 to 40 mg s.c. 50 mg i.p.	Analgesic
Phenoxy-benzamine HCl (soln. last for weeks, it is dissolve in 95% ethanol containing 0.001 ml of 0 N) HCl/ml)	Rat Mouse	1 mg i.v. 10 to 20 mg i.p.	α-Adrenoceptor blocker neuronal and extraneuronal CA uptake blocker; 2 hrs. before experiment
Phentolamine mesylate or HCl	Rat	10 mg i.v.	α–Adrenoceptor blocker 30 min. before test
	Mouse	10 mg i.p.	
Phenylbutazone	Rat	100 to 600 mg p.o 200 mg s.c.	Anti-inflammatory agent

Table 1 *Contd*

Drugs	Animals	Dose per kg body weight and route	Effects & Remarks
A	B	C	D
Sodium salicylate (soln. lasts for weeks)	Rat	500 mg i.p.	Anti-inflammatory
Sotalol	Rat	10 mg i,v.	β_1- Adrenoceptor blocker
Spiroperidol (dissolve in a few drops glacial acetic acid and then distilled water added, pH6)	Rat Mouse	2 to 4 mg i.p. 0.1 mg i.p.	DA antagonist; 20 mins, before experiment
Streptozotocin (dissolve in ice cold 50 mM sodium citrate buffer pH 4.5)	Rat Mouse	35 to 55 mg i.v. 125 to 150 mg i.v.	Destroys cells of the islets of Langerhans; use after 2 weeks. Use after 7 days
Succinylcholine choride	Rat	450 μg i.v	Depolarizing neuromuscular blocker
Sulpiride	Rat	0.1 mg i.v.	DA antagonist
Tetrabenazine methane	Rat	25 mg s.c,	5-HT depletory; 6 hrs, prior to experiment.
Sulfonate	Mouse	30 mg s.c.	
Tolazoline HCl	Rat	10 mg i.p.	α-Adrenoceptor blocker.
Tremorine dihydro-chloride	Rat Mouse	5 to 20 mg i.p./s.c./i.m.	Tremoorgenic
Trifluo-perazine HCl	Rat	10 to 100 mg s.c.	To induce catalepsy
Trimethadione	Rat	40 mg s.c.	Antiepileptic
Tripelennamine HCl	Rat	10 mg i.v.	H_1-Receptor antagonist
U-14624	Rat	200 mg i.p.	Central depletion of NA more than peripheral.
Yohimbine HCl	Rat	1 mg i.p.	Presynaptic α-receptor blocker;1 hr. before experiment
	Mouse	1 mg i.p.	15 min. before experiment

Based on "Fundamentals of Experimental Pharmacology"

– by M. N. Ghosh

Table 2 Doses of Anaesthetics used for Laboratory Mice and Rats

Name of the anaesthetic	Animal	Solvent & strength	Dose (per kg) Mode of administration	Comments
A	**B**	**C**	**D**	**E**
Chloralose	Rat	10% in propylene glycol	80 mg, i. p., i.v. injection	Chloralose is a safe anaesthetic in nearly all instance.
Urathane	Rat	25% aq. soln.	1.25-1.75 i.m. or s.c. injection	Dose is exceedingly variable usually slowly injected to effect.
Nitrous oxide	Rat	with oxygen (4 : 1) with halothane	3-4% through anaesthetic machine	If higher concentration of halothane are used respiration may be depressed prolong use can cause cardiac arrhythmias.
Sodium Pentobarbitone	Rat Mouse	Dissolved in 10 % alcholol 0.6% soln.	35 mg – i.v. 45-60 -i.p. 35-i.v. 50-60-i.p. 80-p.o	Supplements of 5 mg/kg i.v. as needed during experiment. Slowly injected to deep anaesthesia in about 15 mins. and duration 1-2 hrs.

Table 2 *Contd...*

Name of the anaesthetic	Animal	Solvent & strength	Dose (per kg) Mode of administration	Comments
A	B	C	D	E
Triopental	Rat Mouse		47 mg- i.v. 25 mg-i.v. 50 mg-i.p.	
Ether	Rat	Concentrated	Sufficient quantity by open drop mask	Ether can cause excessive bronchial secretion, but it can safely be used if the animal is injected with astropine (1 mg/kg) before the anaesthesia is induced. Ether will often stop the heart before it stop respiration and condition of animal should be watch closely.
Chloralose & Sodium Pentobarbitone	Rat	Aq. Solution	Chloralose 100-120 mg & Pentobarbitone 30 mg i.v. injection	Can be safely used.
Urethane & Sodium Pentobarbiton	Rat	Aq. Solution	Urethane 400-500 mg & Pentobarbitone 5-20 mg i.p.	Can be safely used.

Table 3 Drugs Concentrations Used for Isolated Preparations of Mice and Rats

Drugs (Mol. Wt.)	Tissue Preparation	Concentration *of drugs (Molar)	Effect
A	B	C	D
Acetylcholine chloride (181.7)	Rat, stomach (fundus) Ieum Caecum Anococcygeus Vas deferens Mouse ileum	10^{-7} to 10^{-4} 10^{-8} to 10^{-7} 2×10^{-8} to 4×10^{-5} 10^{-6} to 10^{-1} 10^{-7} to 10^{-3} 2×10^{-8} to 2×10^{-4}	Muscarinic agonist
Adenosine triphosphate (507.2)	Rat, duodenum Vas deferens	10^{-6} to 10^{-5} 10^{-5}	Purinergic agonist
Adrenaline bitartrate (333.3)	Rat uterus	10^{-8} to 10^{-6}	Adrenoceptor agonist.
Angiotensin II amide (1031.2)	Rat, uterus ascending colon	10^{-9} to 10^{-7} 2×10^{-9}	Spasmogen.
Apomorphine HCl (312.8)	Rat vas deferens	10^{-8} to 10^{-6}	Dopamine agonist.
Atropine sulphate (694.8)	Rat, anococcygeus caecum stomach strip vas deference mouse vas deferens	10^{-9} to 10^{-6} 10^{-8} to 10^{-7} 10^{-7} 3.4×10^{-6} 3×10^{-5}	Mascarinic agonist.
Bradykinin (1060.2)	Rat duodenum	10^{-10} to 10^{-8}	Relaxant.
Bretylium tosylate (414.4)	Rat, mesenteric artery deferns vas deferns	2×10^{-5} 2×10^{-5}	Adrenergic neurone blocker
Burimamide (212.3)	Rat, uterus Vas deferens	2×10^{-5} to 2×10^{-4} 2.4×10^{-5}	H_2 – receptor antagonist
Carbachol (182.6)	Rat, caecum Uterus	2×10^{-8} to 2×10^{-6} 3×10^{-6} to 5×10^{-6}	Cholinergic Agonist

Drugs (Mol. Wt.)	Tissue Prepation	Concentration of drugs (Molar)	Effect
A	B	C	D
Cimetidine (252.3)	Rat stomach	10^{-4} to 10^{-3}	H_2- Receptor Antagonist
Clonidine HCl (266.6)	Rat, thoracic aorta vas deferens	4×10^{-8} 10^{-10} to 10^{-6}	α_2- Adrenoceptor agonist
Cocaine HCl (339.8)	Rat vas deferens	1.8×10^{-5}	Neuronal catecholamine uptake inhihibitor.
Cyproheptadine HCl (350.9)	Rat anococcygeus	10^{-6}	Serotonin antagonist
Desipramine (302.8)	Rat vas deferns	10^{-7}	Neuronal catecholamine uptake inhibitor.
Desoxycorti costerone acetate (372.5)	Rat heart	3×10^{-5}	Extraneural catecholamine uptake inhibitor
1. 1-dimethyl-4-phenyl piperazinium iodide (DMPP) (318.2)	Rat vas deferens	10^{-7} to 10^{-4}	Ganglionic stimulant
Diphenhydramin e HCl (291.8)	Rat stomach strip	7×10^{-7}	H_1 Receptor antagonist
Dopamine HCl (189.6)	Rat vas deferens	10^{-8} to 10^{-6}	Inhibition of electrical contraction,
Ergometrine maleate (441.5)	Rat uterus	1.1×10^{-1} to 1.1×10^{-3}	Oxytocic agent.
Guanethidine sulphate (494.7)	Rat vas deferens	10^{-6} to 10^{-5}	Adrenergic neuron blocker
Haloperidol (375.9)	Rat vas deferens	10^{-10} to 10^{-8}	Dopamine antagonist
Hexamethonium bromide (362.2)	Rat, vas deferens anococcygeus	10^{-6} 10^{-4}	Ganglion blocker
Histamine acid phosphate (352.2)	Rat vas deferens	10^{-7} to 10^{-4}	H-Receptor agonist.
5-Hydroxyl-tryptamine creatinine sulphate (5HT serotonin)	Rat, vas deferens anococcygeus fundus caecum	10^{-7} to 10^{-5} 10^{-7} to 10^{-5} 10^{-8} to 10^{-5} 10^{-8} to 10^{-5}	Tryptaminergic agonist

Table 3 *Contd...*

Drugs (Mol. Wt.)	Tissue Prepation	Concentration of drugs (Molar)	Effect
A	B	C	D
Imipramine HCl (316.9)	Rat anococcygeus	10^{-6}	Neuronal catecholamine uptake inhibitor.
Indomethacin (357.8)	Rat, vas deferens urinary bladder	1.4×10 5×10^{-6}	Prostaglandin synthetase inhibitor.
Iproniazid phosphate	Rat splenic strips	3.6×10^{-4}	MAO inhibitor
Isoprenaline HCl, sulphate (556.6)	Rat, vas deferens uterus anococcygeus caecum	3.5×10^{-6} 5×10^{-7} 10^{-6} 3×10^{-9} to 10^{-7}	- Adrenoceptor agonist.
Methoxamine HCl (247.7)	Rat mesentaric artery	4×10^{-6} to 4×10^{-5}	α_1- Adrenoceptor agonist
Methysergide bimaleate (469.5)	Rat, vas deferens anococcygeus stomach strip ascending colon	2.8×10^{-7} 2×10^{-8} to 10^{-6} 6×10^{-7} 10^{-7}	Serotonin antagonist
Morphine HCl (375.8)	Mouse vas deferens	10^{-8}	Inhibits electrical contraction
Naloxone HCl (363.8)	Mouse vas deferens	10^{-7} to 10^{-6}	Opiate antagonist
Neostigmine bromide (303.2)	Rat anococcygeus	10^{-6}	Cholinoceptor agonist
Nialamide (298.3)	Rat anococcygeus	2.2×10^{-6}	MAO inhibitor
Nifedipine (346.3)	Rat vas deferens thoracic aorta	10^{-6} 10^{-7}	Calcium antagonist.
Noradrena (Norepinephrine) Bitartrate (337.3)	Rat, thoracic aorta and portal vein, vas deferens uterus Uterus Caecum Mesenteric artery	10^{-11} to 10^{-6} 10^{-8} to 10^{-4} 10^{-6} 10^{-8} to 10^{-7} 10^{-7}	α - Adrenoceptor agonist

Table 3 *Contd...*

Drugs (Mol. Wt.)	Tissue Prepation	Concentration of drugs (Molar)	Effect
A	**B**	**C**	**D**
Oxprenolol HCl (301.8)	Rat ascending colon	3 3 × 10^{-5}	α – Adrenocepter blocker
Oxytocin (1007.2)	Rat uterus	2 × 10^{-9} to 2 × 10^{-8}	Oxytocic
Papaverine HCl (375.8)	Rat uterus	3 × 10^{-6}	Smooth muscle relaxant
Phenoxy benzamine strip HCl (340.3)	Rat splenic	10^{-6}	Neuronal catecholamine uptake inhibitor.
Phentolamine mesylate (377.5)	Rat, anoccocygeus uterus Vas deferens caecum stomach strip	1^{-8} to 10^{-6} 5 × 10^{-7} 3.5 × 10^{-6} 10^{-7} to 10^{-5} 7 × 10^{-7}	α -Adrenoceptor blocker
1-Phenylephrine (203.7)	Rat thoracic aorta	3 × 10^{-8}	α–Adrenoceptor agonist
Physostigmine or Eserine salicylate (413.4) sulphate (648.8)	Rat caecum	8 × 10^{-7}	Cholinoceptor agonist
Pimozide (416.6)	Rat vas deferens	4 × 10^{-9} to 2.5 × 10^{-7}	Dopamine antagonist
Polyphloretin Phosphate	Rat, uterus ascending colon	10 to 50 μg/ml 20 μg/ml	Prostaglandin antagonist
Potassium chloride (74.6)	Rat mesenteric artery Mouse, ileum vas deferens	10^{-3} to 1.5 × 10^{-2} 4 × 10^{-3} 4 × 10^{-3}	Spasmogen
Prazosin HCl (419.9)	at, vas deferens thoracic aorta	2 × 10^{-5} 10^{-10} to 10^{-9}	α_1 – Adrenoceptor blocker
d, 1-Propranolol HCl (295.8)	Rat, caecum splenic strip uterus vas deferens stomach strip	10^{-7} to 10^{-6} 1.7 × 10^{-6} 10^{-6} 1.9 × 10^{-7} 7 × 10^{-5}	α_1– Adrenoceptor blocker
Prostaglandin E_2 (352.5)	Rat, mesenteric artery uterus aorta	10^{-8} to 3 × 10 9 × 10^{-5} 9 × 10^{-4}	Contraction

Table 3 *Contd...*

Drugs (Mol. Wt.)	Tissue Prepation	Concentration of drugs (Molar)	Effect
A	B	C	D
Prostaglandin F_2 α (354.5)	Rat, mesenteric artery Aorta	10^{-5} 3×10^{-5}	Contraction
Pyrogallol (126.1)	Rat anococcygeus	2.3×10^{-5}	Catechol-O-methyl-transferase (COMT) blocker
SC-19220 (33.0)	Rat stomach	5×10^{-5}	PG-Receptor antagonist
Tetrodotoxin anhydrous (319.3)	Rat anococcygeus	2×10^{-7}	Inhibition of axonal conduction
d-Tubocurarine chloride (771.7)	Rat phrenic nerve diaphragm	10^{-6} to 10^{-4}	Neuromuscular blocker
Verapamil HCl (491.1)	Rat, thoracic aorta & portal vein fundus	10^{-7} to 10^{-6} 10^{-6} to 10^{-5}	Calcium antagonist
Yohimbine HCl (390.9)	Rat, vas deferens thoracic aorta	10^{-7} to 10^{-5} 5×10^{-8} to 10^{-7}	α - Adrenoceptor blocker

Based on "Fundamentals of Experimental Pharmacology"

– by M. N. Ghosh.

Table 4 Sensitivity of different isolated tissue of laboratory rats preparations to some biologically active substances

Preparations	5-HT	ACh	AT	BK	NA	A	H
Rat ascending colon	20×10^{-7} (C)	2.0×10^{-8} (C)	2.0×10^{-6} (C)	2.0×10^{-7} (R)	2.0×10^{-7} (R)	2.0×10^{-7} (R)	10^{-5} (C)
Rat stomach strip	10^{-9} (C)	2.0×10^{-9} (C)	2.0×10^{-9} (C)	2.0×10^{-8} (CorR)	2.0×10^{-7} (R)	2.0×10^{-7} (R)	0
Rat duodenum	20×10^{-8} (C)	2.0×10^{-7} (C)	2.0×10^{-7} (C)	2.0×10^{-9} (R)	2.0×10^{-7} (R)	2.0×10^{-7} (R)	0 0

5-HT – 5-Hydroxytryptamine
A Ch – Acetylcholine
AT – Angiotensin
BK – Bradykinin
NA – Noradrenaline
N – Adrenaline
H – Histamine

Based on "Fundamentals of Experimental Pharmacology" – by M.N. Ghosh,

Table 5 Composition of some physiologic salt solution used for isolated tissue preparations of laboratory Mice and Rats**

Composition of Salts	Ringer or Ringer Locke (Locke)	De Jalon	Tyrode	Krebs Henseleit (Krebs)	Mc Ewen	Mukovic
A	B	C	D	E	F	G
NaCl (58.45)	154(9.0) *	154(9.0)	137(8.0)	118(6.9)	113(7.6)	113(6.6)
KCl (74.56)	5.6 (0.42)	5.6(0.42)	2.7(0.2)	4.7(0.35)	5.6(0.42)	4.6(0.34)
$CaCl_2$ (110.99)	2.2(0.24)	0.55(0.06)	1.8(0.2)	2.5(0.28)	2.2(0.24)	2.5(0.28)
$MgCl_2$ (95.23)	–	–	0.1-1.0	–	–	–
$MgSO_4$ $7H_2O$ (246.39)	–	–	–	1.2(0.28)	–	1.1(0.26)
$NaHCO_3$ (84.00)	6.0(0.5)	6.0(0.5)	11.9(1.0)	25.0(2.1)	25.0(2.1)	25.0(2.1)
NaH_2PO_4 (119.97)	–	–	0.4(0.5)	–	1.2(0.16)	–
KH_2PO_4 (136.08)	–	–	–	1.2(0.16)	–	1.1(0.15)
Glucose (180.16)	5.55(1.0) or 11.1(2.0)	2.78(0.5)	5.55(1.0)	5.55(1.0) or 11.1(2.0)	11.1(2.0)	11.1(2.0)
Sucrose (342.31)	–	–	–	–	13.1(4.5)	–

Values in parentheses indicate mol. wt. of salts * Values are in mM(g/1).

** All salt solutions should be prepared with fresh glass-distilled water and the reagents must all be of analytical grade.

– pH of the salt solutions varies usually between 7.3-7.4.

– Temperature of the bath solutions should be maintained at a specific level.

– Air, O_2 or O_2 + 5% CO_2 is needed for proper functioning of the tissue

Based on "Fundamentals of Experimental Pharmacology"– by M.N Ghosh.

Table 6 Experimental Details for some common isolated Preparations of Laboratory Mice & Rats of tissues

Tissue preparation	Perfusion fluid used	Tempe-rature (O_c)	Gas used	Lever type	Tension (gms)	Magni-fication used
A	B	C	D	E	F	G
Rat						
Ileum or duodenum	Dejalon	30-31	O_2 or 5% CO_2 in O_2	Isotonic frontal	0.5	15
Ileum ascending colon	Tyrode Krebs	37 37	O_2 5% CO_2 in O_2	Isotonic frontal Isotonic frontal	0.25 2	7 4
Descending colon	DeJalon	25	O_2 or 5% CO_2 in O_2	Isotonic frontal	2	4
Stomach (fundus)	Tyrode	37	O_2	Isotonic frontal	1	5-16
	DeJalon or Krebs	37	5% CO_2 in O_2	Isotonic frontal	1	5-16
Anococcygeus	Krebs	36 or 37	5% CO_2 in O_2	Isotonic frontal	0.2-1	10
Uterus	DeJalon	25 to 36	O_2 or 5% CO_2 in O_2 in O_2	Isotonic frontal	0.5-1	4
	Krebs	37	5% CO_2 in O_2	Isotonic frontal	4	4
	McEwen	34	O_2	Isotonic frontal	4	4
	Locke	37	5% CO_2 in O_2	Isotonic frontal	4	10
Vas deferens	Krebs Henseleit Ringer Tyrode	37 37 32	5% CO_2 in O_2 Air 5% CO_2 in O_2	Isotonic Forntal Isotonic frontal	0.5-1 0 5 1	6 6-8 6
	Mc Ewen	32 or 37	5% CO_2 in O_2	Isotonic frontal	0.35	6
Phrenic nerve-diaphragm	Tyrode (double glucose or Krebs)	31 or 37	O_2 or 5% CO_2 in O_2	Spring loaded or simple		8-18

Table 6 *Contd...*

Tissue preparation	Perfusion fluid used	Tempe-rature (O_c)	Gas used	Lever type	Tension (gms)	Magni-fication used
A	B	C	D	E	F	G
Mouse						
Ileum	Ringer	37	Air	Isoronic frontal	0.2	6-8
Vas deferens	Ringer Krebs	37 37	Air 5% CO_2	Isotonic frontal Isotonic frontal	0.2 0.5-1	6-8 0.1-1
	Hukovic	32	5% CO_2	Isotonic frontal	0.3	10-15

Based on "Fundamentals of Experimental Pharmocology".

– by M.N. Ghosh.

GUIDELINES FOR CARE AND USE OF ANIMALS IN RESEARCH

1. Housing, caring, breeding and maintenance of experimental animals to keep them in physical comfort and good health and to permit them to grow, reproduce and behave normally.
2. Sources of experimental animals of known genetic, health and nutritional status.
3. Development of training facilities for scientists, technicians and other supportive staff for the care of animals and their use in experiments.
4. Acceptable experimental techniques and procedures for anesthesia and euthanasia.
5. Developing alternate *in-vitro* systems to replace animal experiments.
6. The constitution of institutional ethics committees, their functions and the legal and ethical obligations to ensure minimal and ethical use of animals.

Sources of Experimental Animals

Authentic source of animals for research should be from recognized scientific animal facilities where the animal colonies of known genetic and health status are available.

Laboratory Animal Husbandry and Management

1. Housing and Environment

   The cages should be made of suitable metal (stainless steel, galvanized iron sheet/rods) or synthetic material (polypropylene/polycarbonate) and of suitable size for each species of animal and should have adequate arrangement for feeding and watering.

   Common bedding materials used such as paddy husk saw dust, paper currings, and dry grass and crushed corn cobs.

2. Nutrition and Feeding

   Only quality ingredients should be used in a diet and they should be free from dust, moulds, fungi and other contaminants.

3. Hygience and Disease Control

A regular medical checkup of the staff, postmortem of dead and sacrificed animals and screening of waste material of the rooms are essential.

Transport of Laboratory Animals

The main considerations for transport of animals are, the mode of transport, the containers, the animal density in cages, food and water during transit, protection from transit infections, injuries and stress.

Anaesthesia

1. Local Anaesthesia: Local anaesthetics are used to block the nerve supply to a limited area and are used only for minor and rapid procedures. This should be carried out under expert supervision for regional infiltration of a surgical site, nerve blocks and for epidural and spinal anaesthesia.
2. General Anaesthesia: A number of agents are used as inhalants. General anaesthetics are also used in the form of intravenous or intra-muscular injections such as barbiturates. Species characteristics and variation must be kept in mind where using an anaesthetic. Side-effects such as excessive salivation, convulsions, excitement and disorientation should be suitably prevented and controlled.

Euthanasia

Euthanasia means "easy death". The procedure should be carried out quickly and painlessly is an atmosphere free from fear or anxiety. A number of euthanasia methods have been recognized humane which could be physical, use of inhalant gases, injectable drugs and general anaesthetics in heavy dose.

Disposal of Animal Carcasses

All animal carcasses whether healthy, infectious or radioactive, must be packed in polythene bags before sending them for disposal. All healthy or infectious animals may be buried deep in the ground covered with lime and disinfectants or burnt in an incinerator.

Laboratory Animal Ethics

The Head of the Institution, maintaining animals for scientific experiments, should constitute an Animal Ethics Committee for experimentation to ensure that all experiments conducted on animals are rational, do not cause undue pain or suffering to the animals

An Animal Ethics Committee should include: a senior biological scientist of the Institute, two scientists from different biological disciplines, a veterinarian involved in care of animals, the scientist incharge of animal facility, a scientist from outside the institute, a non-scientific socially aware member and a member or nominee of appropriate regulatory authority of Govt. of India.

Ethical Guidelines for Use of Animals in Scientific Research

1. Animal experiments should be undertaken only after due consideration of their relevance for human or animal health and the advancement of knowledge.
2. The animals selected for experiment should be of an appropriate species and quality, and minimum number should be used to obtain scientifically and statistically valid results.
3. Investigators and other personnel should treat animals with kindness and should take proper care by avoiding or minimizing discomfort, distress or pain.
4. Investigators should assume that all procedures which would cause pain in human beings may cause pain in other vertebrate species also (although more needs to be known about the perception of pain in animals).
5. Procedures that may cause more than momentary pain or distress should be performed with appropriate sedation, analgesia or anaesthesia in accordance with accepted veterinary practice. Surgical or other painful procedures should not be performed on unanaesthetized animals.
6. At the end of, or when appropriate during an experiment, the animal that would otherwise suffer severe or chronic pain, distress, discomfort, or disablement that cannot be relieved or repaired should be painlessly killed under anaesthesia.
7. The best possible living condition should be provided to animals used for research purpose. Normally the care of animals should be under the supervision of a veterinarian or a person having adequate experience in laboratory animal care.
8. It is the responsibility of the investigator to ensure that personnel conducting experiment on animals possess appropriate qualifications or experience for conducting the required procedures. Adequate opportunities have to be provided by the institution for inservice training for scientific and technical staff in this respect.
9. *In-vitro* systems to replace or reduce the number of animals should be used wherever possible.

GOOD LABORATORY PRACTICES (GLP) FOR ANIMAL RESEARCH

This is for researchers, like you, on the necessities of the FDA's Good Laboratory Practices (GLP) regulations in research studies using laboratory animals. These regulations are appropriate to any animal studies for which results will be used to sustain applications for research or marketing permits for products regulated by the FDA. Such products include human and animal drugs or food additives, medical devices for human use, or biological products. GLPs apply to studies aimed at establishing the safety of drugs or devices, not to basic exploratory, mechanism of action, or efficacy studies. GLP certification was established by the regulatory bodies to ensure that research submitted to them is not only properly executed, but is also documented thoroughly enough so that any scientist skilled in the art can follow the documentation and replicate the results. The level of detail required to achieve this level of documentation is substantial — so much so that the cost of generating the documentation exceeds the cost of the research itself. GLPs are complex and require strict adherence for compliance with standards. Detailed standard operating procedures and record keeping are required for all aspects of the study. Good Laboratory Practice (GLP) embodies a set of principles that provides a framework within which laboratory studies are planned, performed, monitored, recorded, reported and archived. These studies are undertaken to generate data by which the ***hazards and risks*** to users, consumers and third parties, including the environment, can be assessed for pharmaceuticals, agrochemicals, veterinary medicines, industrial chemicals, cosmetics, food and feed additives and biocides. GLP helps assure regulatory authorities that the data submitted are a true reflection of the results obtained during the study and can therefore ***be relied upon when making risk/safety assessments***.

GLP compliance requires the following

- A **Study Director**, appointed by the institution, who acts as the single source of study control and assures that the protocol is approved and followed, that all experimental data are recorded, that GLPs are followed, and that all raw data, documentation, protocols, specimens, and final reports are archived as required.

- An independent **Quality Assurance Unit** that assures management that facilities, personnel, practices and records are in compliance with regulations, maintains a master schedule sheet of studies, inspects each nonclinical study at intervals to assure compliance and report's findings to the Study Director and management, reviews the final report to assure that it accurately reflects the raw data, and prepares and signs a QA statement in the final report.
- **Standard Operating Procedures(SOP)** for equipment use, maintenance, and calibration; for laboratory tests and methods; animal use issues such as identification, care, transfer, and necropsy; histopathology; handling test and control articles; data handling and storage. Any deviations from these SOPs must be authorized and recorded by the Study Director.
- A **written protocol for each study** that describes the objectives and methods for the conduct of the study.
- **Final report** containing a compliance statement signed by the applicant, the sponsor, and the study director.

GLP in Preclinical Research

The role of GLP studies in drug discovery is confusing to many scientists. The confusion has two causes.

- **Semantic:** GLP is an acronym for "Good Laboratory Practices." Hence, many scientists infer that GLP studies must therefore be "good" and non-GLP studies are of questionable quality. Actually, the "good" is more about good documentation than good science.
- **Regulatory requirements:** The regulatory bodies require GLP for far fewer types of studies than many scientists think. GLP requirements are for safety studies, not other types of studies.

The consequences of this confusion are that many drug-discovery organizations end up wasting time and resources on unnecessary and premature GLP studies when their objectives would be better achieved without the burden of GLP.

Animal House Facility

To minimize the effects of environmental variables on the animal, the facility should be designed and operated to control selected parameters (such as temperature, humidity and light). In addition, the facility should be organized in a way that prevents the animals from coming into contact with disease, or with a test item other than the one under investigation. Requirements will be different depending upon the nature and duration of the studies being performed in the facility. Risks of contamination can be reduced by a "barrier" system, where all supplies, staff and services cross the barrier in a controlled way.

A typical animal house should have separations maintained by provision of areas for:

- Different species and for different studies
- Quarantine area
- Changing rooms
- Receipt of materials
- Storage of materials
  - Bedding and diet,
  - Test doses
  - Cages
  - Cleaning equipment
- Necropsy
- Waste disposal

Animal House

1. The building and rooms of animal house should provide sufficient space for animals and studies, allowing the operators to work efficiently.
2. The environment control system should maintain the temperature, humidity and airflow constantly at the defined levels for the species concerned.
3. Design should allow easy and thorough cleaning of surfaces of walls, doors, floors and ceilings. There should be no gaps or ledges where dirt and dust can accumulate. Water should not accumulate on uneven floors i.e. floors should be smooth and even and without crevices.
4. Environmental factors controlled and/or measured: Temperature / humidity, Air flow, Light (intensity and duration), Noise
5. Cleaning: Smooth flat surfaces, walls, doors, ceilings, No gaps, cracks, holes.

Facilities in animal house

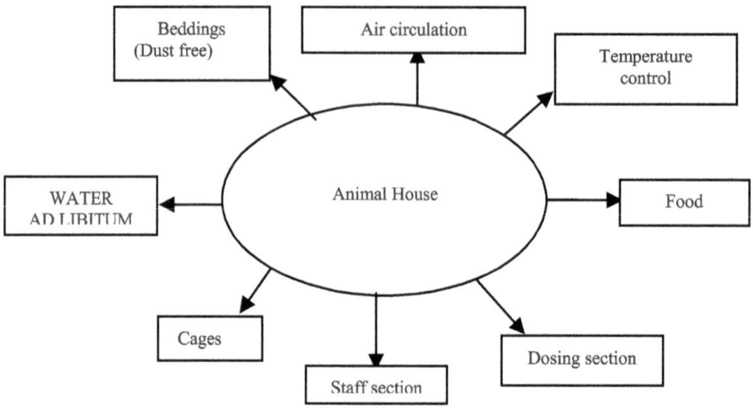

When to Use GLP

GLP is unnecessary until the final stage of preclinical development, at which point GLP documentation is needed for obtaining regulatory approval for further development. Many researchers are under the mistaken impression that at the IND (Investigational New Drug) stage all studies must have GLP documentation. Actually, the FDA requires GLP documentation for **only safety studies**. This includes animal toxicity, genotoxicity, supporting toxicokinetic studies, and safety pharmacology.

GLP is **NOT** required for:

- Efficacy studies, whether *in vitro* or *in vivo*. In fact, the IND application has no requirement at all for mechanism of action or efficacy studies.
- *In vitro* studies, including:
  - Pharmacokinetic analyses that support the *in vivo* efficacy and toxicity studies
  - Drug-drug interaction studies[3]
  - *In vitro* ADME studies

The reasons for this are easy to understand. At the IND stage the regulators' key concern is about toxicity from exposure to the New Chemical Entity (NCE). Their goal is to ensure safety for human subjects. Other risks, such as whether the NCE is efficacious or has drug-like ADME properties are essentially commercial risks that are the responsibility of the filer. In fact, safety is core to the definition of GLP:

Inappropriate Application of GLP

For the types of studies where the regulators do not require GLP, many scientists mistakenly believe that GLP is better than non-GLP. However, at the discovery stage GLP has profound disadvantages, making it unsuitable for discovery-stage work.

- **Inflexibility**
  In the early stages of drug discovery large uncertainties exists about how to conduct experiments. New information is constantly being generated, causing frequent changes in experimental design. Under GLP, every step taken must be decided and documented in advance, and each study must then be scheduled.
- **Pace**
  Because of the documentation burden, GLP studies take 4-5 times longer to execute.
- **Cost**
  All of that documentation makes the cost of GLP 2-10 times greater, depending on the complexity of the study.
- **Scientific challenge**

  The most skilled and creative scientists do not work in GLP environments, as the work is not only repetitive, but mostly paperwork rather than conducting experiments and discussing scientific implications to move the program forward.

GLP and Discovery Research

Research approaches that are optimal at the discovery stage are different from those required for regulatory filings. To provide the needed flexibility, discovery work is best performed by highly experienced and trained scientists who know how to recognize and address the unusual and unexpected outcomes that are the norm during discovery. Because the path to success at the discovery stage is through the process of failing fast, failing cheap, and failing often, the optimal discovery research methodology focuses on the fastest and most cost-effective methods for getting correct scientific answers to direct further research.

The documentation needs of a discovery team are different from the documentation needs of regulators. Regulators need to be able to follow the research without prior background. They need protocols recorded in great detail such that someone with no prior involvement in the research can replicate the experiments if needed. Discovery teams embody substantial organization knowledge. They just need the essentials of the actual research — the key details and the implications — and the assurance that the research is scientifically valid (e.g., that controls and calibration standards were run for each assay, etc.).

Avoiding Surprises

Regulatory filings are goal for any discovery team. Every team wishes to ensure that their filings present a strong case. Well-disciplined teams do this by replicating every study they file to ensure it is all correct. If GLP is required, GLP is utilized to replicate work originally performed non-GLP. If GLP is not required, replicating the study under GLP just adds to the cost of filing.

REFERENCES

References

Abrams, G.D. et al (1963). *Lab. Invest.,* 12, 355.

Adams, W. S. et al (1945). *Amer. J. Physiol.,* 144, 297,

Albrechat, W. et al (1956). *Z. Natorforsch.,* 11b, 248.

Albright, F. (1933). *N. Engl. J. Med.,* 209, 476.

Alho. A. (1961). *Acta. Pathol. Microbiol. Scand ;* Suppl., 149, l.

Altman, J. and Das, G. D. (1966). *J.Camp. Neurol.,* 126, 237.

Altmann, G.G. and Enesco, M. (1967). *Amer. J. Anat.,* 120. 319,

Altman, P.L. and Katz, D.D. (1979). *Biological Hand Books III, Inbred and Genetically Defined Strains of Laboratory Animals Part I : Mouse and Rat,* Federation of American Societies for Experimental Biology, Bethesda, U.S.A.

Altman P.C. and Dorothy, D. *Biology DATA Book* (2nd Ed), Federation of American Society for Experimental Biology, Bethesda Maryland, U.S.A.

Animal Welfare Institute (1958). *Basic Care of Experimental Animal,* Animal Welfare Institute, New York.

Arnesen. K. (1963). *Acta. Pethol. Microbiol. Scand.,* 58, 212.

Annis, D. (1962). *Ann. Ray, Coll. Surg. Engl.,* 31, 23.

Andrew, G.S. (1951), *J. Anat.,* 85, 44.

Anonymons (1970). *Nature* (London), 226, 869.

Andreasen, E. and Christen Sen, S. (1949). *Anat. Rec.,* 103, 401.

Arai, H. (1920). *Amer. J. Anat.,* 28, 59.

Arey, L.B. (1954). *Developmental Anatomy* (6th Ed.), W.B. Saunders, Phliadelphia

Arrington, L.R. (1978). *Introductory Laboratory Animal Science,* The Breeding Care and Management of Experimental Animals (2nd Ed.). The Inter State Printers and Publishers, Inc-Illinois.

Asdell, S.A. (1946). *Patterns of Mammalian Reproduction,* Comstock, Ithaca.

Bailey, P.C. et al (1970). *J. Nat. Cancer Inst.,* 45, 59.

Baker, H. J., Lindsey, J. R. and Weisbroth, S.H. (1980). *The Laboratory Rat, Vol. I-Biology and Diseases,* Academic Press Inc-London-New York.

Baker, H. J., Lindsey, J. R. and Weisbroth, S. H. (1980). *The Laboratory Rat, Vol II -Research Applications*, Academic Press-London - New York.

Barnett, S. A. (1966). *The Rat : A Study in Behaviour* (3rd Ed.) Aldine Publishing Co., Chicago.

Bass. B. G. and Buckley, N. M. (1996). *Amer. J. Physiol.*, 210, 854.

Bell, G.H. (1959). Experimental Physiology, Livingstone. Edinburgh.

Benirschke, K. Garner, F. M. and Jones, T. C. (1978). *Pathology of Laboratory Animals.* Vol - II, Springer-Verlag, New York-Heidelberg-Berlin.

Benirschke, K. Garner F.M. and Jones, T. C. (1978). *Pathology of Laboratory Animals.* Vol-II, Springer-Verlag, New York-Heidelberg Berlin.

Bhalla, T. N. and Bhargava, K. P. (1980). *J. Pharmacol Meth.*, 3, 9.

Bianchi, C. and Franceschini, G. (1954) *Br. J. Pharmac. Chemother*, 9, 280.

Biddle, F. G. and Petras, M. L. (1967). *Genetics.*, 7, 943.

Bielschomsky, M, . et a1 (1939). *Proc. Univ. Otago Med. Sch.*, 37, 9.

Bielschowsk, M. and Bielschowsky. F. (1953). *Proc. Univ. Otago Med. Sch.*, 31, 29.

Bielschowsky, M. et a1 (1956). *Brit. J. Cancer*, 10, 688.

Bielschowsky, M. and Schofield G. C. (1962). *Aust. J. Exp. Biol. Med. Sci.*, 40, 395.

Bockme, B. H. (1967). J. Reticuloendothel. Soc., 4, 438.

Bielschowsky, M. et a1 (1968) *Ibid.,* 48, 54.

Bielschowsky, M. and Goodwall C. M. (1970*) Cancer Res*. 30, 834.

Boyd, E. M. (1942). *J. Biol. Chem.*, 143, 131.

Boyse, E, A. et a1 (1968). *Proc. Ray Soc.*, B170, 175,

Braverman, P. M. (1968). *J. Invest. Dermatol.*, 50, 483.

Burns, B.D. (1961). *Methods in Medical Research*, Ed-in-Chief,

Quastel, J. H ; Vol. 9, P. 347, Year Book Medical Publishers, Inc. Chicago.

Bragdon, J. H ; et al (1957), *Proc. Soc. Exp. Biol. Med.*, 95, 282.

Brezenoff, H. E. (1973), *Brit., J. Pharmacol.*, 49, 565.

Cass, J.S. (1971). *Laboratory Animals : An Annotated Bibliography of Informational Resources, Covering Medicine Science (including Husbandry Technology*), Hafner Publishing Company-New York.

Chatterjee, T.K. et al (1992). *Ind. J. Expt. Biol.*, 30, 839.

Chevrel, M.L. et al (1967). *Bull. Cancer*, 54, 7.

Coates, M.E., O' Donoghue P. N., Payne, P. R. and Ward, R. T. (1969). *Laboratory Animal Hand Books, No. 2-Dietary Standards for Rats and Mice*, Laboratory Animals Ltd.-London.

Cohen, B.L. and Shreffler, D. C. (1961). *Genet Res.*, 2 30 6.

Cole, W.H. (1944). *Ibid.,* 147, 165.

Colley, R. K. and Vanderwolf, C.H. (1978). *Stereotoxic Surgery in the Rat. A Photographic Series* (2nd Ed.), A. J. Cirby and Co-Ontario.

Comline, R. S. and Silvoc, M. (1970). *J. Physiol.*, (London), 209, 587.

Conalty, M. L. (1967) *Husbandry of Laboratory Animals*, Academic Press-London and New York.

Cooke, R. E. et al (1952). *J. Clin. Invest* , 31, 1006.

Cook, M. J. (1965). *The Anatomy of the Laboratory Moose*, Academic Press-London and New York.

Cotchin, E. and Roe, F. J. C. (1967). *Pathology of Laboratory Rats and Mice*, Blackwell Scientific Publications- Oxford and Edinburg.

Crispens, C. G. Jr. (1975). *Handbook on the Laboratory Mouse*, Charles C. Thomas Publishers-Springfield, Illinois.

D' Amour, F. E. and Smith, D. L. (1974). *J. Phrmac. Exp. Ther.*, 72, 14.

D' Amour, F. E. and Blood, F. R. (1959). *Manual for Laboratory work in Mammalian Physiology*, The University of Chicago Press-Chicago.

Danaldson, H. H. (1924). *The Rat, Memories of the Wistar Institute of Anatomy and Biology*, No. 6-Philadelphia.

Delorenzo, R. J. and Ruddle, F. H. (1969). *Biochem. Genet.*, 3, 151.

Delorenzo, R. J. and Ruddle. F. H. (1970). *Ibid,* 4, 259.

Denton, D, A. et al (1952) *Acta. Med. Scand, Suppl.,* 261.

D'onovan, G. E. (1953). *Medical Electronics*, Bulterworth-London.

Eddy, N. B. and Leimbach, D. (1953). *J. Pharmac Exp. Ther.*, 107, 305.

Eggen, D. A. et al (1969). *Ann. N. Y. Acad. Sci.*, 162, 110.

Farris, E. J. (1950) *The care and Breeding of Laboratory Animals*, John Wiley and Sons-New York.

Farris, E. J. and Griffith, J. O. (1949). *The Rat in Laboratory Investigation* (2nd Ed.), J. P. Lippincott, Philadelphia, Pa.

Felligrino, L. J. Cushman, A. J. (1967). *A Stereotaxic Atlas of rat brain-I*, Allan Memorial Institute, McGill University-Montreal, Canada.

Festing, M. F. W. (1979). *Inbred Strains in Biomedical Research*, Macmillan Press Ltd.-London.

Flynn, R. J. (1973). *Parasites of Laboratory Animals*, Iowa State University Press-Iowa.

Fogh, J. and Giovanella, B.C. (1978). *The Nude Mouse in Experimental and Chemical Research*. Academic Press-New York, San Francisco and London.

Ford-Hutchinson, A, W., Smith, M. J. H., Ellion, P.N.C.

Bolam, J. P., Walker, J. R. Lobo, A. A. ; Babcock, J. H.

Colledge, A.J. and Billimoria, F. J. (1975). *J. Pharm. Pharmac.*, 27, 106.

Forter, G, and Lane-Petter, W. (1962). *Notes for Breeders of Common Laboratory Animal*, Academic Press-London and New York.

Fresting, M.F.W. (1979). *Inbred Strains in Biomedical Research*, Macmillan Press-London.

Fukuhara, M. and Tsurufuji, S. (1969). *Biochem, Pharmac.*, 18, 475.

Fukawa, K.; Kawano, O. ; Hibi, M. ; Misaki, N. ; Ohba, S. and Hatanaka, T. (1980). *J. Pharmacol. Meth.*, 4, 251.

Garton, G.A. and Duncan, W.R.H. (1964). *Biochem. J.*, 92, 472.

Ghosh, M. N. ; Banerjee, R. M. and Mukherji, S. K. (1963). *Ind. J. Physiol. Pharmacol.*, 7, 17.

Ghosh, M.N, and Singh, H. (1974). *Br. J. Pharmac.*, 51,503.

Ghosh, M. N. (1984). *Fundamentals of Experimental Pharmacology*, Scientific Book Agency, Calcutta.

Graham- Jones, Ed, (1964). *Small Animal Anaesthesia*, Pergamon- -Oxford.

Greene, E.C. (1935). *Anatomy of the Rat*, Hafner Publishing Cornpany -New York.

Greene, E. L. (1966). *Biology of the Laboratory Mouse* (2nd Ed.), McGraw-Hill Book Company-New York,Toronto, Sidney and London.

Grunberg, H. (1952). The Genetics of the Mouse (2nd Ed.), Martinas Nijhoff -The Hague and London.

Hafez, E.S.E. (1970). *Reproduction and Breeding Techniques for Laboratory Animals*, Lee and Febiger-Philadelphia.

Harkness, J. E. and Wagner, J. E. (1977). The Biology and Medicine of Rabbits and Rodents, Lee and Febiger-Philadelphia.

Hayashi, G. and Takemori, A. E. (1971). *Eur. J. Pharmac.*, 16, 63.

Hebel R. and Stormberg. M. W. (1976). *Anatomy of the Rat*, The Williams and Wilkins Co.-Baltimore.

Herrlein, H.G. (1949). *A Practical Guide on the Care of Small Animals for Medical Research*, Rock land Farms, New City (Rock land Country)-New York.

Hodges, R. D. (1965). *Unpublished*, Wye College. Univ.-London.

Institute of Laboratory Animal Resources,-National Academy of Sciences-Notional Research Council (1967). *Standards for the Breeding Care and Management of Laboratory Rats*, National Research Council, National Academy of Sciences, Washington.

Institute of Laboratory Animal Resources, NRC-NAS, USA (1969). *Procurement Specification VII Rodents*. ILAR Sub-Committee on Rodent and Rabbit Procurement Standards. National Research Council- National Academy of Sciences-Washington.

Institute of Laboratory Animal Resources, NRC-NAS, USA (1971).

A Guide to Infections Diseases of Mice and Rats, National Research Council Academy of Sciences-Washington.

Institute of Laboratory Animal Resources, NRC -NAS, USA (1973).

Procurement Specification. IX. Defined Laboratory Rodents and Rabbits, ILAR Sub-committee on Defined Rodents and Rabbits. National Research Council-Nation 1 Academy of Sciences-Washington.

Institute of Laboratory Animal Resources,–National Academy of Sciences, National Research Council, Assembly of Life Sciences, Division of Biological Sciences, Institute of Laboratory Animal Resources (1976). *Spontaneously Hypertensive (SHR) Rats* :

Guidelines for Breeding, Care and use, National Academy of Sciences-Washington.

Institute of Laboratory Animal Resource, NRC -NAS, USA (1976).

Long term Holding of Laboratory Rodent; ILAR Committee on Long Term Holding of Laboratory Rodents National Research Council-National Academy of Sciences-Washington.

Institute of Laboratory Animal Resources, NRC - NAS, USA (1977).

Laboratory Animal Management-Rodents, ILAR Committee on Rodents. National Research Council-National Academy of Sciences - Washington.

Kolatkar, S. B. Kulkarni, S. D. and Joglekar, G. V. (1973). *Ind. J. Pharmacol*,, 5, 378.

Konig J. F. R., Klippel, E. A. (1963). *The rat brain: A Stereotoxic Atlas of Forebrain and Lower parts of Brain System*, Williams and Wilkins Co.-Baltimore, Maryland.

LAIS Centre News, (1980-'82). National Institute of Nutrition,-Hyderabad.

Lambert, R. (1965). *Surgery of the Digestive System in the Rats*, Charles C. Thomas-Springfield Illinois.

Lane-Petter, W, (1961). *Provision of Laboratory Animals for Research*, Elsevier Publishing Company-Amsterdam,-London. New York and Princeton.

Lane-Petteer, W. (1963) *Animals for Research -Principles of Breeding and Management.* Academic Press-London and New York.

Lane-Petter, W. and Pearson, A. E. G. (1971). *The Laboratory Animals, -Principles and Practice*, Academic Press Inc-New York.

Littlejohn, A. (1996). *Res. Vet. Sci*., 10, 263.

Lumb, W. V. (1963). *Small Animal Anaesthesia*, Lee and Febiger-Philadelphia.

McSherry, B. J. and Grinyer. J. (1954). *Amer. J. Vet. Res*., 15, 509.

Meir, R., Schuler, W. and D'esaulles, P. (1950). *Experientia*, 6, 469.

Melby, E. C. Jr. and *Allanan*, N. H. (1974). *Handbook of Laboratory Animal Science*, Vol, I, CRC Press-Cleveland and Ohio.

Melby, E. C. Jr. and Altman, N. H. (1974). *Handbook of Laboratory Animal Science*, Vol. II, CRC Press-Cleveland and Ohio.

Melby, E. C. Jr. and Altman, N. H. (1976). *Handbook of Laboratory Animal Science*, Vol. III, CRC Press-Cleveland and Ohio.

Mitruka, B. M. ; Rawnsley, H. M. and Vadhera, D. V. (1976). *Animals for Medical Research, Models for the Study of Human Disease*, John Wiley and Sons-New York, London, Sydney and Toronto.

Mitrukt, B. M. and Rownsley H. M. (1977). *Clinical Biochemical and Hematological Reference Values in Normal Experimental Animals*, Abacus Press Ltd.-Tun Bridge Wells.

Morse, III H. C. (1978). *Origins of Inbred Mice*, Academic Press-New York, San Francisco and London.

Munson, E. S. et al (1970). *J. Appl. Physiol.*, 28, 108.

Mulbock, O. (1976). Proceedings of the *Workshop on Basic Aspects of Freeze Preservation of Mouse Strains*, Gustav Fischer Verlag- Stuttgart.

National Academy of Sciences (1971). *Defining the Laboratory Animal,* IV. Symposium, International Committee on Laboratory Animals.

National Academy of Sciences- Washington.

National Academy of Sciences, National Research Council, Institute of Laboratory Animal Resources (1976). *Guide for the Care and use of the Nude (Thymus-deficient) Mouse in Biomedical Research*, Washington National Academy of Sciences, National Research Council, USA (1978)

Nutrient Requirement of Laboratory Animals (3rd Ed.), National Academy of Sciences-Washington.

Newbould, B. B. (1963). *Br. J. Pharmac. Chemother.*, 21, 127.

Olmested. F. and Page, I. H. (1966). *Amer. J. Physiol.*, 210, 817,

Orlans, B. F. (1977). *Animal Care from Protozoa to Small Mammals* Addison Wesley Publishing Co., Menlopark, C.A. ; USA.

Owen, D. (1972). *MRC Laboratory Animals Centre Handbooks-: No. L Common Parasites of Laboratory Rodents and Lagomorphs*, Her Majesty's Stationary Office-London.

Parmer, N. S. and Ghosh, M.N. (1978). *Ind. J. Pharmacol.* 10 277.

Paton, W. D. M. (1957). *J. Physiol.*, 137, 35.

Proter, G. and Lane-Petter, W. (1962). *Notes for Breeders of Common Laboratory Animals*, Academic Press -London and New York.

Raiser, R. et al (1959). *Circ. Res.*, **7**, 833.

Richard, L. Dofy. (1976). *Mammalian Olfaction, Reproductive Process and Behaviour*, Academic Press-New York, San Francisco and London.

Roberts, D. C. (1969). Laboratory Animal Handbook. No 3: *Transplanted Tumours of Rats and Mice. An Index of Tumours and Host Strains*, Laboratory Animals Ltd.-London,

Rabinson, R. (1965). *The Genetics of the Norway Rat*, Pergamon Press-Edinburgh, Frankfurt, London, New York, Oxford and Paris.

Rowsell, H. C. et al (1960). *Can. Med. Ass. J.* 83, 1175.

Rossodale, P. D., and Mullen P. A. (1970). *Brit. Vet. J.*, 126, 82.

Rowett, H. G. O. (1957). *The Rat as a small Mammal*, John Murray, Fifty Albemarle Street, London.

Rugh, R. (1968). *The Mouse-Its Reproduction and Development*, Burgess Publishing Company-Minneapolis.

Rygward, J. and Povlsen, C. O. (1974). *Proceedings of the First International Workshop on Nude Mice*, Custav Fischer Verlag-Stuttgart.

Rygward, J. and Povlsen, C. O. (1977). *Bibliography of the Nude Mouse* (1966-1970), Gustav. Fischer Verlag-Stuttgart and New York,

Selye, H. (1953). *Proc. Soc. Exp. Biol. Med.*, 82, 328.

Short, D. J. and Woodnott, D.P. (1969). *The IAT Manual of Laboratory Animal Practice and Techniques* (2nd Ed.), Crosby Lockwood-London.

Smith, E. M. and Calheun, M. L. (1968). *The Microscopic Anatomy of the white Rat*, Iowa State University Press-Ames and Iowa.

Simmons, M. L. and Brick, J. O. (1970). *The Laboratory Mouse: Selection and Management*, Prentice Hall-Englewood cliffs and New Jersey.

Smith, M. J. H., Ford-Hutchinson, A. W., Elliot, P. N. C. and Bolam J.P (1974). *J. Pharm. Pharmac.*, 26, 692.

Singh, H. and Ghosh. M. N. (1968). *J. Pharm. Pharmac.*, 20, 316.

Sofia, R. D., Knoblock, L. C, and Vassar, H, B. (1975). *J. Pharmac. Exp. Ther.*, 193, 918,

Srivastava (1974). *The Vertebrate Types (Frog and Rat)*, Oxford and IBH Publishing Co.-New Delhi, Bombay and Calcutta.

Staff of the Deptt. of Pharmacology, University of Edinburgh (1970). *Pharmacological Experiments on Isolated and Intact Preparations,* Churchill Livingstone-Edinburgh, London and New York.

Strozier, L. M. et al. (1971). *Lab. Anim. Sci.*, 21, 399.

Swenson, M. J. ed. (1970). *Dukes Physiology of Domestic Animals*, (8th Ed.). Cornell Univ. Press. Ithaca. P-52.

The USAP School of Aerospace Medicine (1966). *Selected Topics in Laboratory Animal Medicine Series-Vol. XIV : The Mouse*, Brooks Air Force Base, National Technical Information Service, 5285 Port Royal Road, Springfield VA 22161.

Theiler. K. (1972). *The House Mouse-Development and Normal* Stages *from Fertilization to* 4 *Weeks* of *age*, Springer Verlag-Berlin, Heidelberg and New York,

Turner, A. R. (1965). *Screening Methods in Pharmacology*, Academic Press-New York and London.

Turusov, V, S. (1976). *Pathology of Tumours in Laboratory Animals. Vol.* I. *Tumours of the Rat. Part 2*, Lyon. Intrenational Agency for Research on Cancer.

United States Department of Agriculture (1968). *Raising Mice and Rats for Laboratory use.* Leaflet No, 483, U. S. Govt Printing Office Washington.

Walker, D. G., Wirtschafter, Z. T. (1957). *The Genesis of the Rat Skeleton : A Laboratory Atlas*, Charles C. Thomas-Sprinfield Illinois.

Wells, T. A. S. (1968). *The Rat: A Practical Guide*, Heinemane Educational-London.

Whitehouse, M. W. (1965). *In Progress in Drug Research*, Vol. 8, Jucker, E. Birkhouser Verlag - Basel.

Williams, C. S. F. (1976). *Practical Guide to Laboratory Animals*, The C. V. Mosby Company-Saint Louis.

Winter, C. A., Risely, E. A. and Nuss, G. W. (1962). *Proc. Soc.* Exp. *Biol. Med.,* III, 544.

UFAW Staff (1976). *The UFAW Handbook on the Care and Management of Laboratory Animals* (5th.Ed.), Churchill Livingstone-New York.

Vinegar, R., Truax, J. F. and Selph, J. L. (1973). *Proc. Soc. exp. Biol. Med.* 143, 711.

Zeman, W. and Maitland Innes J. R. (1963). *Craigie's Neuroanatomy of the Rat*, Academic Press-New York and London.

APPENDIX

Appendix

Table of Profits*

%	0	1	2	3	4	5	6	7	8	9
0	-	2.67	2.95	3.12	3.25	3.36	3.45	3.52	3.59	3.66
10	3.72	3.77	3.82	3.87	3.92	3.96	4.01	4.05	4.08	4.12
20	4.16	4.19	4.23	4.26	4.29	4.33	4.36	4.39	4.42	4.45
30	4.48	4.50	4.53	4.56	4.59	4.61	4.64	4.67	4.69	4.72
40	4.75	4.77	4.80	4.82	4.85	4.87	4.90	4.92	4.95	4.97
50	5.00	5.03	5.05	5.08	5.10	5.13	5.15	5.18	5.20	5.23
60	5.25	5.28	5.31	5.33	5.36	5.39	5.41	5.44	5.47	5.50
70	5.52	5.55	5.58	5.16	5.64	5.67	5.71	5.74	5.77	5.81
80	5.84	5.88	5.92	5.95	5.99	6.04	6.08	6.13	6.18	6.23
90	6.28	6.34	6.41	6.48	6.55	6.64	6.75	6.88	7.05	7.33

Table of distribution of t*

			Probability			
DF	***0.5***	***0.1***	***0.05***	***0.02***	***0.01***	***0.001***
A	*B*	*C*	*D*	*E*	*F*	*G*
1	*1.000*	*6.314*	*12.706*	*31.821*	*63.657*	*636.619*
2	*0.816*	*2.920*	*4.303*	*6.965*	*9.925*	*31.598*
3	*0.765*	*2.353*	*3.182*	*4.541*	*5.841*	*12.941*
4	*0.741*	*2.132*	*2.776*	*3.747*	*4.604*	*8.610*
5	*0.727*	*2.015*	*2.571*	*3.365*	*4.032*	*6.859*
6	*0.718*	*1.943*	*2.447*	*3.143*	*3.707*	*5.959*

Table *Contd...*

Probability						
DF	***0.5***	***0.1***	***0.05***	***0.02***	***0.01***	***0.001***
A	***B***	***C***	***D***	***E***	***F***	***G***
7	*0.711*	*1.895*	*2.365*	*2.998*	*3.499*	*5.405*
8	*0.706*	*1.860*	*2.306*	*2.896*	*3.355*	*5.041*
9	*0.703*	*1.833*	*2.262*	*2.821*	*3.250*	*4.781*
10	*0.700*	*1.812*	*2.228*	*2.764*	*3.169*	*4.587*
11	*0.697*	*1.796*	*2.201*	*2.718*	*3.106*	*4.437*
12	*0.695*	*1.782*	*2.179*	*2.681*	*3.055*	*4.318*
13	*0.694*	*1.771*	*2.160*	*2.650*	*3.012*	*4.221*
14	*0.692*	*1.761*	*2.145*	*2.624*	*2.977*	*4.140*
15	*0.691*	*1.753*	*2.131*	*2.602*	*2.947*	*4.073*
16	*0.690*	*1.746*	*2.120*	*2.583*	*2.921*	*4.015*
17	*0.689*	*1.740*	*2.110*	*2.567*	*2.898*	*3.965*
18	*0.688*	*1.734*	*2.101*	*2.552*	*2.878*	*3.922*
19	*0.688*	*1.729*	*2.093*	*2.539*	*2.861*	*3.883*
20	*0.687*	*1.725*	*2.086*	*2.528*	*2.845*	*3.850*
21	*0.686*	*1.721*	*2.080*	*2.518*	*2.831*	*3.819*
22	*0.686*	*1.717*	*2.074*	*2.508*	*2.819*	*3.792*
23	*0.685*	*1.714*	*2.069*	*2.500*	*2.807*	*3.767*
24	*0.685*	*1.711*	*2.064*	*2.492*	*2.797*	*3.745*
25	*0.684*	*1.708*	*2.060*	*2.485*	*2.787*	*3.725*
26	*0.684*	*1.706*	*2.056*	*2.479*	*2.779*	*3.707*
27	*0.684*	*1.703*	*2.052*	*2.473*	*2.771*	*3.690*
28	*0.683*	*1.701*	*2.048*	*2.467*	*2.763*	*3.674*
29	*0.683*	*1.699*	*2.045*	*2.462*	*2.756*	*3.659*
30	*0.683*	*1.697*	*2.042*	*2.457*	*2.750*	*3.646*
40	*0.681*	*1.684*	*2.021*	*2.423*	*2.704*	*3.551*
60	*0.679*	*1.671*	*2.000*	*2.390*	*2.660*	*3.460*
120	*0.677*	*1.658*	*1.980*	*2.358*	*2.617*	*3.373*
α	*0.674*	*1.645*	*1.960*	*2.326*	*2.576*	*3.291*

Table of Wilcoxon test on unpaired samples* 5% Critical points of rank sums

$n_1 \rightarrow$	2	3	4	5	6	7	8	9	10	11	12	13	14	15
$n_2 \downarrow$														
4			10											
5		6	11	17										
6		7	12	18	26									
7		7	13	20	27	36								
8	3	8	14	21	29	38	49							
9	3	8	15	22	31	40	51	63						
10	3	9	15	23	32	42	53	65	78					
11	4	9	16	24	34	44	55	68	81	96				
12	4	10	17	26	35	46	58	71	85	99	115			
13	4	10	18	27	37	48	60	73	88	103	119	137		
14	4	11	19	28	38	50	63	76	91	106	123	141	160	
15	4	11	20	29	40	52	65	79	94	110	127	145	164	185
16	4	12	21	31	42	54	67	82	97	114	131	150	169	
17	5	12	21	32	43	56	70	84	110	117	135	154		
18	5	13	22	33	45	58	72	87	103	121	139			
19	5	13	23	34	46	60	74	90	107	124				
20	5	14	24	35	48	62	77	93	110					
21	6	14	25	37	50	64	79	95						
22	6	15	26	38	51	66	82							
23	6	15	27	39	53	68								
24	6	16	28	40	55									
25	6	16	28	42										
26	7	17	29											
27	7	17												
28	7													

1% Critical points of rank sums

$n_1 \rightarrow$	2	3	4	5	6	7	8	9	10	11	12	13	14	15
$n_2 \downarrow$														
5				15										
6			10	16	23									
7			10	17	24	32								
8			11	17	25	34	43							
9		6	11	18	26	35	45	56						
10		6	12	19	27	37	47	58	71					
11		6	12	20	28	38	49	61	74	87				
12		7	13	21	30	40	51	63	76	90	106			
13		7	14	22	31	41	53	65	79	93	109	125		
14		7	14	22	32	43	54	67	81	96	112	129	147	
15		8	15	23	33	44	56	70	84	99	115	133	151	171
16		8	15	24	34	46	58	72	86	102	119	137	155	
17		8	16	25	36	47	60	74	89	105	122	140		
18		8	16	26	37	49	62	76	92	108	125			
19	3	9	17	27	38	50	64	78	94	111				
20	3	9	18	28	39	52	66	81	97					
21	3	9	18	29	40	53	68	83						
22	3	10	19	29	42	55	70							
23	3	10	19	30	43	57								
24	3	10	20	31	44									
25	3	11	20	32										
26	3	11	21											
27	4	11												
28	4													

n_1 and n_2 are the number of cases in the two groups. If the groups are unequal in size, n_1 refers to the smaller.

* Based on 'Fundamentals of Experimental Pharmacology'

– by M. N. Ghosh

Weights †

Scale			Table	Grams	Grains
Kilo	–	–	1 Kilogram =	1000.0 =	15,432.85
Hecto	–	–	1 Hectogram =	100.0 =	1,543.23
Deca	–	–	1 Decagram =	10.0 =	154.323
Unit	–	–	1 Gram =	1.0 =	15.482
Deci	–	–	1 Decigram =	0.1 =	1.5432
Centi	–	–	1 Centigram =	0.01 =	0.15432
Milli	–	–	1 Miligram =	0.001 =	0.01543
Micro	–	–	1 Microgram =	10^{-6} =	15.432×10^{-6}
Nano	–	–	1 Nanogram =	10^{-9} =	15.432×10^{-9}
Pico	–	–	1 Picogram =	10^{-12} =	15.432×10^{-12}
Femto	–	–	1 Femtogram =	$10–^{15}$ =	15.432×10^{-15}
Autto	–	–	1 Attogram =	10^{-18} =	15.432×10^{-18}

SI Base Units †

Quantity	Name	Symbol
Length	meter	m
Mass	kilogram	kg
Time	second	s
Electric current	ampere	A
Temperature	kelvin	K
Luminous intensity	candela	cd
Amount of substance	mole	mol

Some SI Derived Units †

Quantity	Name of Derived Unit	Symbol
Area	square meter	m^2
Volume	cubic meter	m^3
Speed, velocity	metter per second	m/s
Acceleration	meter per second squared	m/s^2
Density	kilogram per cubic meter	kg/m^3
Concentration of substances	mole per cubic meter	mol/m^3
Specific volume	cubic meter per kilogram	m^3/kg
Luminescence	candela per square meter	cd/m^2

SI Derived Names with Special Names †

Quantity	Name	Symbol	Expressed in Terms of other Units
Frequency	hertz	Hz	S^{-1}
Force	newton	N	$kg.m.s^{-2}$ or $kg.m/s^{-2}$
Pressure	pascal	Pa	$N.m^{-2}$ or N/m^2
Energy, work, amount of heat	joule	j	N.m
Power	watt	W	j.s or j/s
Quantity of electricity	coulomb	C	A.s
Electromotive force	volt	V	W/A
Capacitance	farad	F	C/V
Electrical resistance	ohm	∩	V/a
Conductance	siemens	S	A/V
Inductance	henry	H	w/A
Illuminance	lux	lx	ln/m^2
Absorbed (radiation) dose	gray	Gy	J/kg

Prefixes and Multiples used in SI †

Prefix	Symbol	Power	Multiple or Portion of a Multiple
tera	T	10^{12}	1,000,000,000,000
giga	G	10^{9}	1,000,000,000
mega	M	10^{6}	1,000,000
kilo	k	10^{3}	1,000
hecto	H	10^{2}	100
deca	da	10^{1}	10
unity			1
deci	D	10^{-1}	0.1
centi	C	10^{-2}	00.1
milli	m	10^{-3}	0.001
micro	µ	10^{-6}	0.000001
nano	N	10^{-9}	0.00000000001
pico	P	10^{-12}	0.0000000000001
femto	F	10^{-15}	0.000000000000001
atto	a	10^{18}	0.0000000000000001

Units of Length †

Millimeters	Centimeters	Inches	Feet	Yards	Meters
1 mm = 1.0	1.0	0.03937	0.00328	0.0011	0.001
1 cm = 10.0	1.0	0.3937	0.03281	0.0109	0.11
1 m = 25.4	2.54	1.0	0.0833	0.0278	0.0254
1 ft = 304.8	30.48	12.0	1.0	0.333	0.3048
1 yd = 914.40	91.440	36.0	3.0	1.0	0.9144
1 m = 1000.0	100.0	39.37	3.2808	1.0936	1.0

1 μ = 1 mu = 1 micrometer = 0.001 millimeter 1 mm = 1000 μ.

1 km = 1 kilometer = 1000 meters = 0.6215 mile.

1 mile = 5280 feet = 1.609 kilometers.

Units of Volume (fluid or liquid) †

Milliliters	U.S. Fluid Drams	Cubic Inches	U.S. Fluid Ounces	U.S. Fluid Quarts	Liters
1 ml = 1.0	0.2705	0.061	0.03381	0.00106	0.001
1 fl 5 = 3.697	1.0	0.226	0.125	0.00391	0.00369
1 cu In = 16.3866	4.4329	1.0	0.5541	0.0173	0.01639
1 fl 3 = 29.573	8.0	1.8047	1.0	0.03125	0.02957
1 qt = 946.332	256.0	57.75	32.0	1.0	0.9463
1 L = 1000.0	270.52	61.025	33.815	1.0567	1.0

1 gallon = 4 quarts = 8 pints = 3.785 liters

1 pint = 473.16 ml

Units of Weight †

Grians	Grams	Apothecaries Ounces	Avoirdupis Pounds	Kilograms
1 gr. = 1.0	0.0648	0.00208	0.0001429	0.000065
1 gm. = 15.432	1.0	0.03215	0.002205	0.001
1 g. = 480.0	31.1	1.0	0.06855	0.0311
1 lb. = 7000.0	453.5924	14.583	1.0	0.45354
1 kg = 15432.358	1000.0	32.45	2.2046	1.0

1 γ = 1 gamma = 1 microgram = 0.001 milligram ; 1000 γ = 1 mg

1 mg = 1 milligram = 0.001 gm ; 1000 mg = 1 gm

1 grain = 64.8 mg ; = 1 mg = 0.0154 grain

Weight and Measures †

Apothecaries Weight

20 grains = 1 scruple	3 scruples = 1 dram
8 drams = 1 ounce	12 ounces = 1 pound

Avoiredupois Weight

27.343 grains = 1 dram	16 drams = 1 ounce
16 ounce = 1 pound	100 pounds = 1 hundred weight
2000 pounds = 1 short ton	2240 pounds = 1 long ton
1 oz troy = 480 grains	1 oz avoirdupois = 437.5 grains
1 lb troy = 5760 grains	1 lb avoirdupois = 7000 grains

Circular Measure

60 seconds = 1 minute	60 minutes = 1 degree
90 degrees = 1 quadrant	4 quadrants = 360 degrees = circle

Cubic Measure

1728 cubic inches = 1 cubic foot	27 cubic feet = 1 cubic yard
2150.42 cubic inches = 1 standard bushel	268.8 cubic inches = 1 dry (U.S) gallon
1 cubic foot = about four fifths of a bushel	128 cubic feet 1 = 1 cord (wood)

Dry Measure

2 pints = 1 quart	8 quarts = 1 peck	4 pecks = 1 bushel

Liquid Measure

16 ounces = 1 pint	4 quarts = 1 gallon	2 barrels = 1 hogshead (U.S.)
1000 milliliters = 1 liter	31.5 gallons = 1 barrel (U.S)	1 quart = 0.946 liters
4 gills = 1 pint	2 pints =1 quart	

Barrels and hogsheads vary in size. A.U.S. gallon in equal to 0.8327 British gallon; therefore a British gallon is equal to 1.201 U.S. gallons. 1 liter is equal to 1.0567 quarts.

Linear Measure

1 inch = 2.54 centimeters	40 rods = 1 furlong	8 furlongs = 1 stature mile
12 inches = 1 foot	3 feet = 1 yard	5.5 yards = 1 rod
1 statute mile = 5280 feet	3 statute miles = 1 statute league	

Troy Weight

24 grains = 1 pennyweight; 20 pennyweight = 1 ounce; 12 ounce = 1 pound

Used for weighing gold silver, and jewels

Household Measure* and Weights

Approximate Equivalents : 60 gtt. – teaspoonful = 5 ml.

= 60 minims = 60 grains = 1 dram = $1/9$ ounce

1 teaspoon = $1/8$ fl. oz.; 1 dram	16 tablespoons (liquid) = 1 cup
3 teaspoon = 1 tablespoon	12 tablespoons (dry) = 1 cup
1 tablespoon = ½ fl. oz.; 4 drams	1 cup = 8 fl. oz.

1 tumbler or glass = 8 fl. Oz. ; ½ pint

* Household measures are not precise. For instance, household tsp will hold from 3 to 5 ml of liquid substances. Therefore, do not substitute household equivalents for medication prescribed by the physician.

Conversion Rules †

In convert units of one system into the other, multiply the number of units in column I by the equivalent factor opposite that unit in column II.

Weight

I		II
1 milligram	=	0.015432 grain
1 gram	=	15.432 grains
1 gram	=	0.25720 apthecaries' dram
1 gram	=	0.03527 avoirdupois ounce
1 gram	=	0.02315 apothecaries' troy ounce
1 kilogram	=	35.274 avoirdupois ounces
1 kilogram	=	32.151 apothecaries' or troy ounces
1 kilogram	=	2.2046 avoirdupois pounds
1 grain	=	64.7989 milligrams
1 grain	=	0.0648 gram
1 apothecaries' dram	=	3.8879 gram
1 avoirdupois ounce	=	28.3495 gram
1 apothecareis' or troy ounce	=	31.1035 gram
1 avoirdupois pound	=	453.5924 gram

Volume (air or gas)

I		II
1 cubic centimeter	=	0.06102 cubic inch
1 cubic meter	=	35.314 cubic feet
1 cubic meter	=	1.3079 cubic yard
1 cubic inch	=	16.3872 cubic centimeters
1 cubic foot	=	0.02832 cubic meter

Capacity (fluid or liquid)

I		II
1 milliliter	=	16.23 minims
1 milliliter	=	0.2705 fluid dram
1 milliliter	=	0.0338 fluid ounce
1 liter	=	33.8148 fluid ounces
1 liter	=	2.1134 pints
1 liter	=	1.0587 quart
1 liter	=	0.2642 gallon
1 fluid dram	=	3.697 milliliters
1 fluid ounces	=	29.573 milliliters
1 pint	=	473.166 milliliters
1 quart	=	946.322 milliliters
1 gallon	=	3.785 liters

To convert Centigrade or Celsius Degrees to Fahrenheit Degress*

Multiply the number of Centigrade degrees by 9/5 and add 32 to the result.

Example ; 55° C × 9/5 = 99 + 32 = 131°F

To convert Fahrenheit degrees and multiply the difference by $\frac{5}{9}$.

Example ; 243°F. – 32 = 211 × $\frac{5}{9}$ = 117.2°C.

Miscellaneous Conversion Factors + Pressure

to obtain	multiply	by
lb. sq. In.	atmosphere	14.696
lb. sp. In.	in of water	0.03609
lb.sq. in	ft. of water	0.4335
lb.sq. in	in of mercury	0.4912
lb.sq. in	kg, sq. meter	0.00142
lb.sq. in	kg. sq. cm	14.22
lb./sq. in.	cm. of mercury	0.1934

Table *Contd...*

lb./sq. ft.	atmospheres	21166.8
lb./sp. ft.	in of water	5.204
lb./sq. ft.	ft. of water	62.48
lb./sq. ft.	in. of mercury	70.727
lb./sq. ft.	cm. of mercury	27.845
lb./sq. ft.	Kg/sq. meter	0.20482
lb./cu. in.	gm./gl.	0.03613
lb./cu. ft.	Lb./cu. in.	1728.0
lb./cu. ft.	gm./ml.	62.428
lb./U.S. gal.	gm./l.	8.345
in. of water	In. a mercury	13.60
in. of water	cm. of mercury	5.3543
ft. of water	atmospheres	33.95
ft. of water	Lb./sq. meter	2.307
ft. of water	Kg./sq. meter	0.00328
ft. of water	in. of mercury	1.133
ft. of water	cm. of mercury	0.4461
atmospheres	ft. of water	0.02947
atmospheres	in. of mercury	0.03342
atmospheres	kg./sq. cm.	0.9678
bars	atmospheres	1.0133
in of mercury	atmospheres	29.921
in of mercury	lb./sq. in	2.036
mm. of mercury	atmospheres	760.0
gm. ml.	lb./cu. in.	27.68
gm.sq. cm	kg./sq. meter	0.1
kg.sq. meter	Lb./sq. in	703.1
kg.sq. meter	In of water	25.40
kg.sq. meter	In of mercury	345.32
kg.sq. meter	cm. of mercury	135.95
kg.sq. meter	atmospheres	10332.0
kg. sq. cm.	atmospheres	10.332

Flow Rate

To obtain	Multiply	By
cu. ft./hr.	cc./min.	0.00212
cu. ft./hr.	L./min	2.12
L. min.	cu. ft./hr.	0.472

Parts Per Million

Conversion of parts per million (ppm) to percent ; 1 ppm = 0.0001%; 10 ppm = 0.001%, 100 ppm = 0.01%, 1000 ppm = 0.1%, 10,000 ppm = 1%, etc.

Miscellaneous Units of Measurement †

Units of Time

1 millisecond = one thousandth (0.001) of a second 1 minute = 1/60 of an hour

1 second = $\frac{1}{60}$ of a minute 1 hour = $\frac{1}{24}$ of a day

Units of Temperature

Given a temperature on the Fahrenheit scale ; to convert it to Centigrade, substract 32 and multiply by 5/9. Given a temperature on the Centigrade scale, to convert it to Fahrenheit, multiply by $\frac{9}{5}$ and 32, Celsius degrees are equivalent to Centigrade degrees.

Units of Energy

1 gram/centimeter = 980.665 dynes/centimeter

1 food-pound = 13,558.200 ergs = 13,825.5 gram-centimeters

1 Joule = 0.2386 Calorie (kilocalorie)

1 Calorie = 4.26649 × 10^7 gram-centimeters = 3085.96 foot-pounds

1 calorie (kilocalorie) = 1000 calories = 4184 Joules

A large Calorie, or kilocalorie, is always written with a capital C.

pH Table

The pH scale is simply a series of numbers stating where a given solution would stand in series of arranged according to acidity or alkalinity, At one extreme (i.e., high pH) lies an alkaline solution made by dissolving 4 gm. of sodium hydroxide in water to make a liter of solution, at the other is a solution containing 3.65gm. of hydrogen chloride per liter. Halfway between lies purified water, which is neutral. All other solutions can be arranged on this scale, and their acidity or alkalinity can be stated by giving the numbers that indicate their relative positions.

Tenth – normal HCl	100
Gastric juice	*14 Litmus is red in
Urine	* 6.0 this acid range
Water	7.0 Neutral
Blood	7.35-7.45
Bile	*75 Litmus is blue in
Pancreatic juice	8.5 this alkaline range
Tenth-normal NaOH	13.00

If one is told that the pH of a certain solution is 5.3 one knows at once that it falls between gastric juice and urine on the above scale, is moderately acid, and will turn litmus red.

* These body fluids very rather widely in pH; typical figures have been used for simplicity. Urine samples obtained from healthy individuals may have pH's anywhere between 4.7 and 8.0.

Preparation of Percentage Solutions

When the metric system is used, the preparation of percentage solutions is simple; a 1% solution contain 1 gm. in 100 ml ; a 0.1% solution contains 0.1 gm. (or 100 milligrams) per 100 ml.

When the apothecaries system is used the following are helpful ; 4.55 grains to the ounce, or 2.5 drams to 32 ounces ; 3.25 drams to 40 ounces ; all make a 1% solution.

To prepare a Dilute Solution from One Which is Stronger

For example, io make 80% alcohol from 95%; Dilute 80 ml. of the 95% alcohol to 95 ml. with distilled water.

Rule ; Dilute a volume equal to the percent desired to a volume equal to the percent used.

† Based on "Taber's Cyclopedic Medical Dictionary" – by C. L. Thomas

INDEX

Index

A

B

C

D

E

F

B

H

I

L

M

N

O

P

Q

R

S

U

V

www.ingramcontent.com/pod-product-compliance
Ingram Content Group UK Ltd.
Pitfield, Milton Keynes, MK11 3LW, UK
UKHW021326190726
13845UKWH00003B/43

9 789385 433511